Coping with Hay Fever

Christine Cr..r in the Civil
Service until..c pain condition. Christi...s, in the past
few years, p..ress. She also
writes for the Fibromyalgia Association UK and the related *FaMily* magazine. In recent years she has become interested in fiction writing, too.

Overcoming Common Problems Series

Selected titles

A full list of titles is available from Sheldon Press,
36 Causton Street, London SW1P 4ST and on our website at
www. sheldonpress.co.uk

The Assertiveness Handbook
Mary Hartley

Assertiveness: Step by Step
Dr Windy Dryden and Daniel Constantinou

Body Language: What You Need to Know
David Cohen

Breaking Free
Carolyn Ainscough and Kay Toon

Calm Down
Paul Hauck

The Candida Diet Book
Karen Brody

Cataract: What You Need to Know
Mark Watts

The Chronic Fatigue Healing Diet
Christine Craggs-Hinton

The Chronic Pain Diet Book
Neville Shone

Cider Vinegar
Margaret Hills

Comfort for Depression
Janet Horwood

**Coming Off Tranquillizers and
Antidepressants**
Professor Malcolm Lader

The Complete Carer's Guide
Bridget McCall

The Confidence Book
Gordon Lamont

Confidence Works
Gladeana McMahon

Coping Successfully with Pain
Neville Shone

Coping Successfully with Panic Attacks
Shirley Trickett

Coping Successfully with Period Problems
Mary-Claire Mason

Coping Successfully with Prostate Cancer
Dr Tom Smith

Coping Successfully with Ulcerative Colitis
Peter Cartwright

Coping Successfully with Varicose Veins
Christine Craggs-Hinton

Coping Successfully with Your Hiatus Hernia
Dr Tom Smith

Coping Successfully with Your Irritable Bowel
Rosemary Nicol

Coping with Age-related Memory Loss
Dr Tom Smith

Coping with Alopecia
Dr Nigel Hunt and Dr Sue McHale

Coping with Blushing
Dr Robert Edelmann

Coping with Bowel Cancer
Dr Tom Smith

Coping with Brain Injury
Maggie Rich

Coping with Candida
Shirley Trickett

Coping with Chemotherapy
Dr Terry Priestman

Coping with Childhood Allergies
Jill Eckersley

Coping with Childhood Asthma
Jill Eckersley

Coping with Chronic Fatigue
Trudie Chalder

Coping with Coeliac Disease
Karen Brody

Coping with Compulsive Eating
Ruth Searle

**Coping with Diabetes in Childhood and
Adolescence**
Dr Philippa Kaye

Coping with Diverticulitis
Peter Cartwright

Coping with Down's Syndrome
Fiona Marshall

Overcoming Common Problems Series

Overcoming Common Problems Series

Overcoming Common Problems

Coping with Hay Fever

CHRISTINE CRAGGS-HINTON

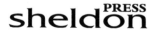

First published in Great Britain in 2008

Sheldon Press
36 Causton Street
London SW1P 4ST

British Library Cataloguing-in-Publication Data

A catalogue record for this book is available from
the British Library

ISBN 978–1–84709–034–8

1 3 5 7 9 10 8 6 4 2

Typeset by Pantek Arts Ltd, Maidstone, Kent
Printed in Great Britain by Ashford Colour Press

Produced on paper from sustainable forests

Contents

Note to the reader

This is not a medical book and is not intended to replace advice from your doctor. Consult your pharmacist or doctor if you believe you have any of the symptoms described, and if you think you might need medical help.

Introduction

Many people look forward to spring, but someone with hay fever comes to dread it, for it literally brings tears to their eyes. Instead of enjoying the blossoming trees and flowers, the beautiful greenery outdoors, hay fever sufferers attempt to stay closeted indoors, fighting a battle against sneezing fits and myriad other cold-like symptoms.

Hay fever is a common condition which can be described as an immune system overreaction to airborne substances such as pollen and mould – substances that a healthy immune system would recognize as 'normal'. Such 'allergens' stimulate the body into producing an excess of the chemical histamine which creates hypersensitivity in the nose, eyes and throat, promoting congestion and excessive mucus production along the way.

Although the causes of hay fever are not fully understood, there is no doubt at all that allergic disease is on the increase – eczema and asthma are closely related to hay fever. One reason for the rise is due to the many challenges today's world presents to the immune system and adrenal glands, such as the number of toxins in the air around us and in the foods we eat. Indeed, the average Western diet is high in processed, prepackaged foods that are full of chemical additives such as flavourings, preservatives and colourings. These weaken the immune system further, making it more sensitive to substances it would ordinarily identify as normal. Stress is also a great presence in western societies and is known to increase the chances of allergic reaction.

Between my teens and thirties, I suffered intermittently from hay fever myself – at times very badly. I well remember the constant sneezing, streaming nose, watering eyes and the way my throat and soft palate used to itch unbearably at times when the pollen count was high. On top of that, I was aware of a kind of nervous irritability, together with a feeling of dull fatigue throughout my body. I also remember the general hypersensitivity I experienced, such as a dislike of loud noises and bright lights, as well as a lowered pain threshold. In addition, being unable to concentrate properly made it impossible for me to do my job as quickly and efficiently as required, so I had no choice but to take time off work. It was a wonderful relief when in my late thirties, the allergy began to loosen its grip and to disappear altogether as I entered my forties.

Although the antihistamines of a few years ago were very good at controlling hay fever symptoms, they were notorious for their sedating effect, and I chose not to take them. Nowadays, however, there is a new type of antihistamine, with all the benefits of the older ones without their tendency to make you feel like a zombie. Other types of treatment currently available can significantly reduce the misery of hay fever, as can the many natural remedies that can be used either in conjunction with chemical medication, or as an alternative. This book discusses all these topics, in addition to dietary recommendations, common-sense advice on getting the most from your life, and many more useful points.

1

Hay fever – an overview

Hay fever is the most common allergy in the Western world, with the number of cases rising annually. In the last 20 years its incidence has actually tripled, which is almost unprecedented for a health disorder. Although studies suggest that hay fever is present in 20 per cent of the population in Western societies, the true figure could be much higher as many individuals attribute their symptoms to a persistent summer cold.

Experts predict the following for the future of hay fever:

- The number of cases will carry on climbing.
- It will continue to emerge in people who have never before suffered from it.

Currently, in the West, it appears that up to 40 per cent of young adolescents suffer the misery of hay fever, as a result of which far too many important school days are lost. Sadly, affected youngsters may not later reach their full potential in their working lives, often causing frustration, low self-esteem and a poorer financial and social status than might otherwise have been. Where adults are concerned, the cost to the exchequer in lost days at work is significant, which is one reason why a great deal of research into hay fever treatments is now under way.

The condition can be described in brief as an immune system reaction (the immune system is the body's natural defence mechanism) to a particular substance – something it mistakenly identifies as an invading force. In hay fever, forms of plant life are recognized as invaders – the pollen from trees, plants, weeds and grasses, together with the fungal spores from different types of mould.

The purpose of the immune system is to attack and destroy invaders. In hay fever, it attempts to fight off a mistakenly identified invader by producing symptoms that mainly affect the nose, sinuses, throat and eyes (see a discussion of the possible symptoms on pages 3–5). The intensity of symptoms can vary from month to month, depending upon the amount of pollen and fungal spores in the air.

Moreover, the type of symptoms can differ from region to region, the determinant factors being the type of allergens circulating in the air at the time and to which substances the individual is allergic. Any substance that is identified by the immune system as an invader is called an *allergen.*

The term *hay fever* is, to some extent, misleading. Although hay is produced from grass, many other plant substances can cause an adverse immune reaction in a susceptible person (the factors that make a person susceptible are explained in Chapter 4). The specific reference to hay is thought to have arisen after early descriptions of sneezing and a streaming nose and eyes while harvesting hay in the field. In fact, it is during the 'haying' season – which generally runs from late May until the end of June – that most plants release their pollen into the air, therefore the allergy reaches its peak during that period.

Hay fever can greatly impact upon a person's general health and overall quality of life. For instance, having a picnic in the countryside on a warm spring day is for most people a pleasurable experience, but someone with hay fever will try to avoid this, particularly when the pollen count is high. Similarly, physical activities such as cycling along tree-lined avenues or playing football on the village green are likely also to be avoided, which is a great shame. Where general health is concerned, it must be said that hay fever can lead to other disorders such as sinusitis, eczema and asthma, which are discussed in Chapter 3.

If you are exhibiting the typical symptoms of hay fever but don't know whether it's actually a cold (which is caused by a viral infection) the timing of your sniffles and sneezes should provide a good clue. As a rule, colds only last for a week or two and usually attack during the cooler months, whereas hay fever symptoms generally last longer and are more likely to be present during the spring and early summer. Moreover, hay fever symptoms often come and go, depending upon the levels of pollen in the air (see 'Likely high pollen times' on pages 14–15).

Hay fever cannot, as yet, be cured, but the symptoms can be controlled. The condition also tends to be far less of a problem as the years go by, peaking during adolescence to mid-twenties and improving or even disappearing as a person reaches their mid-forties. Plenty of other people find, however, that the culprit allergen(s) continues to affect them for a prolonged length of time. Indeed, it may always present symptoms – especially in years when the pollen and mould counts are elevated. Fortunately, the various treatments and self-help measures, as discussed in later pages, can generally reduce the symptoms and allow you to get on with your life.

A minor condition?

People who don't suffer from hay fever may view it as a slightly inconvenient runny nose. For those who do have it, however, the myriad symptoms can make springtime and early summer cripplingly miserable. It is therefore a great deal more than a 'slight' inconvenience, affecting quality of life, causing problems at work and at home and interfering with leisure-time activities. Moreover, when the millions spent on hay fever medications and the cost of lost work days are taken into account, the condition is, without doubt, anything but minor.

You may be interested to know that *allergic rhinitis* – the correct medical term for hay fever – has recently been formally classified as a 'major chronic respiratory disease', which at last adds weight to the condition.

Hay fever symptoms

In the main, hay fever is an allergic reaction to pollen that causes inflammation in the membranes of the following areas:

- the nasal cavities;
- the whites of the eyes;
- the Eustachian tubes (in the ear);
- the middle ear;
- the nasal sinuses (the cavities within the bones and tissues of the face that connect them with the nasal cavities);
- the pharynx (the cavity behind the nose and mouth that connects them with the oesophagus, or gullet).

In hay fever, the nose is always affected, and many individuals experience problems in the other areas mentioned. As a result, sneezing, a runny nose and nasal congestion (see below) occur – the symptoms we all experience when we come down with a cold (the medical term for which is *infective rhinitis*). A cold results from catching a viral infection, whereas hay fever is caused by being allergic to particular pollens, as discussed later in this chapter. A person who is plagued by several allergies, such as to certain foods, household cleaning fluids and/or medications, or has asthma and/or eczema, is far more likely to develop hay fever than a person who is not prone to these things.

The effect of hay fever can vary greatly, some people experiencing mild symptoms and others far more severe. It is not unusual for a person to have mild symptoms that later become far more pronounced, and vice versa.

The symptoms associated with hay fever arise because the immune system of a susceptible person reacts to pollen and moulds as if they are harmful substances – a threat to good health. On reaching the cells that line the mouth, nose, eyes and throat of the person, irritation results, at which a special type of antibody known as immunoglobulin E (IgE) is released into the bloodstream to attack the pollen or mould. IgE then triggers the release of more chemicals, including histamine – and it is this cocktail of chemicals that produces the symptoms of an allergic reaction.

The symptoms that are most commonly linked to hay fever include those listed here.

Itchy nose, mouth, eyes, throat, ears and skin

On contact with pollen, someone with an allergy to it is likely to experience itching in the nose, eyes, throat, roof of the mouth (soft palate), ears and even the skin. Most people with hay fever have itching in just a few of these places, whereas a few have it in them all.

Frequent sneezing

When the mucous membranes – the tissues lining the nose – are irritated by pollen, the body's immediate and automatic response is to try to blow it out. This is the phenomenon we call sneezing.

Streaming nose and eyes

If sneezing is unsuccessful at removing the irritant, the tissues lining the nose start to swell, producing a clear, watery liquid (referred to as *mucus*). The aim of this mucus is to wash out the irritant. In addition, the irritant can cause the eyes to become red, watery and itchy. The watering is the eyes' automatic response to the presence of an irritant and their attempt to remove it. The eyes may also become bloodshot.

The symptoms related to the eyes are combined in the term *allergic conjunctivitis*, which means inflammation of the whites of the eyes.

Blocked nose

When the lining of the nose continues to swell, it begins to block the passage of air and the person has no choice but to breathe through his or her mouth – a situation termed *nasal congestion*. The mucus now also becomes thicker (catarrh) and may also cause earache, headache and the feeling of plugged-up ears.

Coughing

A blocked nose will result in the dripping of mucus down the back of the throat, which in turn causes coughing.

Poor concentration

It is common to experience poor concentration with hay fever – and not only because sore, itchy eyes, a streaming nose and so on are a distraction from what you are trying to do. The symptoms of hay fever can cause irritability and a general feeling of being unwell, which makes it difficult to concentrate.

Listlessness

The presence of hay fever symptoms often causes listlessness and a feeling of being drained.

Disturbed sleep

Hay fever symptoms can make it difficult to get a good night's sleep. It's not unusual to experience poor sleep for several nights in a row, which is likely to lead to further listlessness and fatigue. The blocked nasal passages in hay fever can also cause snoring, which may keep your partner awake!

Less common symptoms

Some of the less common symptoms of hay fever include the following:

- wheezing
- impaired sense of smell
- impaired sense of taste
- face pain (caused by blocked sinuses)
- nose bleeding
- flushing and sweats
- depression
- allergy to some fruits.

Allergic rhinitis

The correct medical term for hay fever is *allergic rhinitis* (or *allergic rhino-conjunctivitis*). For hay fever that emerges during a particular season, such as in high pollen times, the correct term is *seasonal allergic rhinitis* (or *seasonal allergic rhino-conjunctivitis*). However, hay fever that persists throughout the year is termed *perennial allergic rhinitis* (or *perennial allergic rhino-conjunctivitis,* as discussed in the next section). The words 'rhino' and 'rhinitis' are derived from the Greek word for nose – *rhis*. The 'itis' in rhinitis refers to the presence of inflammation.

Allergic rhinitis is actually a blanket term that refers to more than just the pollen allergy that is hay fever. Allergies that produce virtually identical symptoms are included in that term, whatever time of year they are in evidence.

Many people with hay fever are also allergic to the following:

- The microscopic dung pellets from house dust mites. These mites are tiny insects that live in the dust in our homes and are extremely prevalent in our mattresses, in particular. A person who is allergic to house dust mite dung will have year-round symptoms – perennial allergic rhinitis – unless steps are taken to remove or at least reduce the quantity of mites and their dung.
- The mould spores that are produced from fungi. Such spores are often seen in poorly ventilated rooms, particularly in bathrooms – on non-slip bath mats, the inner side of shower curtains and around window frames. For more information on mould, see Chapter 2.
- The dust – called 'animal dander' – produced by the skin of pets and other animals. The feathers in duvets and pillows also create this dust.
- The wool in woollen items such as blankets and knitwear.

Removing hay fever from the equation for a moment, it must be said that the symptoms created by many common allergens – especially those mentioned above – are often worse in winter when the windows and doors in the house are more likely to be kept closed.

Perennial allergic rhinitis

If your sniffles and sneezes seem to be in evidence on low pollen days and in winter, it is likely that you don't have hay fever at all and are suffering from some other kind of allergy or allergies entirely. You should be able to deduce this once and for all by checking out high pollen days and judging whether your symptoms are actually worse on such days. If other allergies are indicated, try to discover your particular allergens and avoid contact with them whenever you can. For instance, a possible allergy to the dung from house dust mites can be assessed by thoroughly beating and vacuuming your mattress to remove most of the mites and their dung. If this is indeed a problem for you, regular vacuuming and turning of your mattress and frequently using freshly laundered bed linen can greatly reduce its adverse effect, as can removing carpets in favour of a different type of floor-covering such as wood, wood-laminate, linoleum and tiles.

Of course, many people with perennial allergic rhinitis are allergic to pollen as well as to other allergens. In addition to pollen, the condition is most commonly caused by repeated contact with any of the following allergens:

- dung from the house dust mite
- animal dander
- indoor mould spores
- certain chemical detergents often used in the home
- an allergy to a particular food.

Perennial allergic rhinitis causes symptoms that are similar to hay fever – that is, the irritation of the delicate mucous membranes that line the upper respiratory tract. If it is possible for you to avoid the culprit allergen, this is your best means of tackling the problem. However, your particular allergens may not be obvious, in which case you would be well advised to speak to your doctor about the possibility of allergy testing.

Who gets hay fever?

In children and adolescents, hay fever is more common in boys than in girls, but this tends to even out as adulthood is reached. The average age of hay fever onset is as young as 8–11 years, with approximately 80 per cent of sufferers developing the condition by 20 years of age.

A person of any race can develop hay fever. However, it is more common among certain populations and cultures. This appears to be due to the following:

- *Genetic factors* – Because hay fever tends to run in families, there would once have been clusters of sufferers in particular regions. As people gained access to wider areas, these clusters would gradually have spread. (Read more about hay fever and genetics in Chapter 4.)
- *Geographical factors* – The pollens that give rise to hay fever are not as prevalent in some parts of the world as in others, therefore there are fewer sufferers in those parts. An obvious example is Greenland, where there are no trees and few grasses. However, in some parts of Switzerland hay fever is rife, with many people having to put up with

symptoms for almost ten months of the year[1] – grass pollen being the chief culprit. In other parts of Switzerland, the length of the hay fever season is no more than two to three months.

- *Environmental factors* – Experts believe that an over-sterile home (and/or workplace), exposure to pollutants such as from smoking, car exhaust fumes and industry, and the use of antibiotics in childhood can make a susceptible person more prone to developing hay fever. (See Chapter 4 for more information on the causes of hay fever.)

Given the right conditions, virtually anyone can develop hay fever. However, individuals in the following groups are more likely than others to develop it:

- people with an inherited tendency, as mentioned;
- firstborn children;
- boys;
- children who have eczema and/or asthma;
- children who have food allergies;
- people with nasal polyps – these are small non-cancerous (benign) growths in the lining of the nose;
- a person (either child or adult) who has other allergies – perhaps to pet fur and dung from the house dust mite;
- a pregnant woman, due to the changes her body is undergoing.

Although the peak age of onset is during adolescence and the twenties, it's not unusual for an elderly person to develop hay fever.

Pollen

In order to take on board how hay fever arises, it is first necessary to have an understanding of what pollen is and how it manages to produce an allergic reaction in some people.

Pollen is composed of dry particles of protein and is produced by many different species of shrubs, grasses and weeds – and also from trees that flower throughout the growing season in the UK. Grasses and flowering trees and plants primarily use air currents – the wind – to transport the male gamete (in effect, the male sex cells which carry genetic self-replicating material, or DNA) to the female part of a neighbouring plant of the same type, with the aim of fertilization. Thousands of microscopic male gametes are encased inside each grain of pollen, which in itself is so tiny it may measure only 15 to 100 microns and appear no larger than the width of an average human hair. Indeed, one pinch of pollen powder will contain many thousands of grains. The outer wall of the grain consists of a very tough substance which protects its cargo on its journey, whereas the inner layer is composed of cellulose – the main constituent of plant cell walls and vegetable fibres. The grain is also very light and dry, enabling it to be carried quite easily on the wind.

Pollen grains are usually invisible in the air. They come in a variety of sizes and shapes that are characteristic of their species, tending to be oval, spherical or disc-shaped. The outer surface of the grain can either be smooth or contain pores, grooves, granulations, spines, furrows or have a meshed appearance. Pollen grains from most grasses, for example, have one pore and no furrows; oak tree pollen contains three furrows and a pore in the centre; and birch tree pollen has three pores and no furrows. Fir trees, pines and spruces give off pollen grains that are winged to enable them to travel further.

The transfer of pollen grains to the female reproductive part of a neighbouring plant is called *pollination* and enables the growth of a new plant with 50 per cent of their genetic make-up from the male part of the initial plant and 50 per cent from the recipient female part of the plant. Some plants are able to self-pollinate, but the majority pollinate with another plant of the same species – a process called *cross-pollination.*

The majority of plants with bright flowers, such as roses, chrysanthemums and daffodils, however, are pollinated by insects, the pollen being relatively heavy, sticky and rich in protein. This attracts insects such as bees to feed on them. In due course, the pollen grains are eliminated from the insect via faeces on to neighbouring same-species plants.

Pollen from flowering plants that attract insects can form into clumps and be visible to the eye, and some people believe this to be the cause of their symptoms. It does indeed have allergenic properties, but as it is comparatively much larger and therefore heavier than wind-borne pollen, there is far less chance of it reaching the nose. Therefore, the chief culprit in triggering hay fever is wind-borne pollen, which issues from the plants listed below.

As mentioned, wind-borne pollen grains are transported by air currents. They waft upwards on the morning breeze and float back down as the ground cools at the end of the day. The reason that hay fever is often worse in the early evening is this increase in numbers of pollen grains in the air around us as they return to earth. They lodge in the nasal mucous membranes and other parts of the respiratory system where they trigger an allergic reaction (see below).

Most species of pollen have allergenic properties, with some being notorious for triggering hay fever symptoms. For example, 60 to 95 per cent of sufferers are affected by grass pollen, whereas around 20 per cent are troubled by birch tree pollen. Approximately 15 species of plants are known to be significantly allergenic and a further five less commonly cause problems. Oak tree and plane tree pollen can be highly allergenic, as can nettle pollen and ragweed (ragweed is an uncommon plant in the UK, but prevalent in the USA, Canada and parts of Europe). To ensure that some pollen reaches its target, plants that use air currents to aid pollination are more likely to produce enormous amounts of pollen, which is another reason why it is likely to be inhaled.

Wind-pollinated plants usually have insignificant flowers that are tiny and greenish-yellow in colour. It is these flowers that produce the pollen.

The exact time that a plant releases its pollen is dependent upon the local climate and the normal 'behaviour pattern' of the plant. As a rule, the further north a plant is, the later in the season it will release its pollen. In contrast to pollen, mould does not have a season and can release its spores at any time of the year. See Chapter 2 for more information on fungal spores.

Hypersensitivity

Until a few decades ago, all types of hypersensitivity were considered to be allergies and believed to be caused by the inappropriate activation of immune system antibodies. These days we know that several different mechanisms are involved in what are now described as 'hypersensitivity reactions', and a new classification has been set up.[2] Under the new classifications, a true allergy is restricted only to 'hypersensitivity reaction type 1', which means that it gives rise to a more severe reaction than in lower classifications of hypersensitivity.

Any hypersensitivity provokes mistaken activation of immune system antibodies, caused by an acquired sensitivity to a substance that would be seen as innocuous to a healthy immune system. Obviously, not all substances set up hypersensitivity reactions, but the ones that do include pollen, dust, yeasts, animal fur, bee venom, house dust mite dung, certain foods and certain drugs.

Allergic reaction

The term 'allergy' was first coined in 1906 by Viennese doctor Clemens von Pirquet, who put together the Greek words *allos* (meaning 'different') and *ergon* ('work'). It is believed he meant that the allergic reaction was caused by something working differently from normal.

As with all hypersensitivity reactions, the culprit substance must gain access to the human body for the backlash to occur. Contact with such a substance can come about in the following ways:

- through the skin
- via lung inhalation
- from touch.

Mounting an attack

People who are not susceptible to allergens experience no adverse reaction after exposure to them. However, inside the body of a person who is susceptible a type of war takes place. Believing it is being invaded by a foreign substance, the body's immune system triggers the production of masses of protective antibodies called *immunoglobulin E* (IgE for short) to mount an attack on the invaders. We all have a number of IgE defenders whose aim it is to fight off invaders, but people who are allergic to certain substances produce too many for their own good when provoked. The result of this sudden overabundance is termed a 'systemic inflammatory response', which means that one of the body's systems – the upper respiratory system, where hay fever is concerned – becomes swollen, reddened, hot and often painful. This response manifests itself as the runny nose, watering eyes and so on that we associate with hay fever.

Allergies to other substances may be so severe that they can result in life-threatening *anaphylactic shock* – an extreme allergic reaction where the blood pressure suddenly drops and there is difficulty breathing. Left untreated, it can even lead to death. Fortunately, an allergy to pollen and the other allergies encompassed in the umbrella term allergic rhinitis is not life-threatening.

There is, as yet, no absolute cure for allergic reactions of any kind. As mentioned earlier, the best treatment of all is avoidance, but this is not always possible.

Being hypersensitive to a substance is not an allergy

Many people still believe that an adverse reaction to a substance – often a type of food – is an allergy. For example, someone who repeatedly suffers an upset stomach the day after eating cheese may say he or she is allergic to cheese, when in fact the problem is actually 'hypersensitivity' (also referred to as intolerance) to cheese. The confusion between the terms allergy and hypersensitivity is still largely in evidence. An allergy is actually limited to the most severe of several grades of hypersensitivity reactions (as mentioned on page 10) and symptoms occur immediately after contact with the allergen, unlike the lower grades of reaction caused by a slow build-up of a problem substance. When a more delayed reaction takes place, the terms we should be using are hypersensitivity or intolerance, rather than allergy.

Food intolerance is always a threat to people who fail to eat a varied diet, for after repeated consumption of a particular food, the body becomes 'sensitized' to it. The result is symptoms ranging from food cravings and stomach irritations (bloating, abdominal cramps and perhaps diarrhoea) to indigestion – all of which are undoubtedly unpleasant. An increasing amount of evidence is prompting experts to believe that irritable bowel syndrome (IBS) develops as a result of food intolerance.

The foods most likely to cause intolerance problems are wheat, corn, food colourings, coffee, yeasts, citrus and dairy products, as well as foods containing chemical additives and preservatives (all processed foods, in effect).

The early stage of a true allergic reaction

In virtually any kind of war, innocent bystanders are affected – and hay fever is no different. The allergic reaction in hay fever gives rise to casualties in special cells called *mast cells*, an injured one of which will immediately release into the bloodstream a cocktail of inflammatory chemicals which includes histamine, tryptase, chymase, kinins and heparin. Before long, additional chemicals such as leukotrienes and prostaglandin D2 flood the bloodstream, interact with the earlier ones and, within minutes, give rise to irritation, itching, swelling and leakage of fluid from the cells, in the form of sneezing, a runny nose and watering eyes.

The late stage of reaction

Within four to eight hours, the above-mentioned chemicals have worked hard to recruit further inflammatory substances, and this results in ongoing inflammation, often extending to wider-ranging mucous membranes. The symptoms produced are similar to those of the early stage, except that there is less itching and sneezing and an increase in congestion and the creation of mucus. The mixture of chemicals can even lead to muscle spasm, which causes tightening in the lungs and throat, such as is present in asthma and laryngitis.

Fatigue, insomnia, irritability and a general feeling of malaise can arise from the late stage of reaction. Accompanying these can be ultra-sensitivity to bright light and loud noise, together with a lowered pain threshold. This invariably has a negative impact on quality of life, at least for the duration of symptoms.

The pollen count

As mentioned earlier, a person with hay fever will normally find that their symptoms worsen when the pollen count is high, and are less in evidence when the count is low. The pollen count is based on the approximate number of pollen grains present in each cubic metre of air, and symptoms are generally produced when the pollen count is over 50. However, some people display symptoms when the pollen count is around 20 grains per cubic metre, whereas others only display them when the count is as high as 100. This is because the body chemistry of every person with hay fever is unique and everyone will have differing levels of sensitivity. Note that during June, the peak pollen time, the pollen count can be as high as 200, which is obviously a great problem for anyone with hay fever.

What affects the pollen count?

The amount of pollen circulating in the air is dependent, first of all, on the weather at the time. For instance, on days that are cloudy, rainy or windless, pollen is less able to move about and so fewer people are troubled with hay fever symptoms. On the other hand, hot, cloudless, dry and windy weather signals more pollen distribution and so allergy symptoms are increased. The amount of pollen in the air during any given season can vary enormously, depending upon variations in temperature and rainfall. These factors may also affect the pollen count from year to year, for as we know only too well in the UK, spring and summer can be surprisingly cloudy and wet, and with the effects of global warming this type of weather may be on the increase.

Would it help to move?

People often think that moving to live in another area, where there are different plants, might reduce their symptoms – but this is not usually the case. As a treatment of hay fever, relocating is not recommended for the following reasons:

- The main allergenic grasses and moulds are present in most plant zones.
- Virtually identical symptoms are likely to be triggered by plants that may look different from the ones you left behind, but are actually related.
- There may be additional allergens from different plants in the new locality and within two years you may find yourself with further allergies.

Instead of moving to a different location in an attempt to lessen your symptoms, it is recommended that you seek the appropriate medical advice and treatment. Following the advice in this book can also be a great help.

The pollen forecast

The pollen forecast is a free service to the public, compiled by aeroallergen counters at some universities, clinics and medical centres. Television, radio and newspaper weather forecasts often give the expected daily pollen count, and it can also be found on many websites. One certified website which gives such details is listed in the Useful addresses section at the back of this book.

Unfortunately, interpreting the pollen and mould counts (see Chapter 2 for information on fungal spores) – assessing the symptoms expected from a particular reading with some degree of accuracy – is not easy for the layperson. It doesn't help that the air sampling equipment used and its location may affect the reading. Moreover, pollen counts can vary enormously from day to day, yet we tend to believe that the readings used are a good indicator. In truth, they are taken between one and three days beforehand and are only a very rough gauge of what might be to come. In short, as a predictor of symptom severity, pollen and mould counts have severe limitations.

It should also be mentioned that hay fever symptoms are likely to temporarily worsen after exposure to another allergen, such as pet dander or a chemical detergent. The timescale of the exposure is also of significance.

Likely high pollen times

Here is the standard hay fever calendar in the UK:

- The pollen season starts in February or March with pollens from trees becoming airborne.

- This is followed, from late May to mid-August, by the pollen from grasses.
- Most weeds pollinate between August and October. It is the low-growing weeds that tend to produce airborne pollen.
- Meanwhile mould, after lying dormant during winter, begins to release its spores into the air in the spring, reaching a peak in July and August and often continuing until the first frost.

Of course, not everyone with hay fever is allergic to all types of pollen. You may be surprised to read, though, that as many as 95 per cent of sufferers are allergic to the pollen from grasses, whereas only 10 per cent are allergic to the pollen from trees. In the USA, approximately 75 per cent of sufferers are allergic to the pollen from ragweed – a plant belonging to the daisy family which produces massive amounts of pollen.

The length of the pollen season has extended in recent years, the pollen count first peaking as early as March. This extension is believed to be another sign of world climate change.

Sources of pollen

In the UK, the following pollens often trigger hay fever symptoms:

- January – alder and hazel
- February – alder, poplar and hazel
- March – elm, poplar, willow, silver birch and ash
- April – silver birch and poplar
- May – grass, horse chestnut, poplar, silver birch, linden and oak
- June – grass, poplar, linden and weeds
- July – grass and weeds
- August – grass and weeds
- September – weeds and fungal spores
- October – fungal spores
- November – fungal spores.

Some people would include oilseed rape for May. However, it is usually the strong-smelling chemicals released by this plant that causes irritation of the upper respiratory tract, as discussed on page 31. The grasses that mostly trigger an allergic reaction include sweet vernal grass, cocksfoot, meadow fescue, common reed, meadow grass, redtop and Johnson grass. The weeds that may provoke hay fever symptoms include nettles and dock.

In the course of a day

As the pollen season gets under way, pollen is released from plants early in the morning. If the day is sunny, more flowers open as the day grows warmer, with their pollen soaring high into the air. The pollen count rises in the early evening, when the air cools and the pollen falls closer to the ground. If the day is windy or humid, pollen tends to travel a greater distance and so pose a problem to more people. On rainy days, pollen is likely to be washed from the air, causing the pollen count to drop.

Hay fever and children

Recent studies have shown a noticeable rise in the incidence of hay fever in children over two years of age, which strongly suggests that at least two seasons of pollen exposure must be experienced for the allergy to develop. This coincides with what we know about allergies – they take more than one exposure to arise.

Research has also shown that children born in spring or early summer are more likely to develop allergies at a younger age than children born at other times of the year. Note, though, that children who wheeze a lot in their first years of life appear to be no more at risk of developing hay fever than those who don't.

Unfortunately, many parents are still being told by doctors that their children are too young to develop an allergy. However, not only can hay fever arise in a toddler, it's also a fact that approximately 15 per cent of children have the condition by their seventh birthday, which is surprisingly young for such a significant incidence rate.

We also know now that children who are in contact with other children from an early age – who attend preschool day nurseries, for example – are less prone to getting hay fever, asthma and other allergies than those who do not. Greater exposure to common viruses would, therefore, seem to allow the immune system to mature, as explained in more detail in Chapter 4.

2

Fungal spores

Moulds, like mushrooms, are types of fungus. They grow on vegetation and animals, examples being alternaria, aspergillus and cladosporium. Their reproductive parts – called *spores* – are transported through the air like pollen, their aim being to find a hospitable environment in which to flourish and grow. However, when these spores – which are invisible to the naked eye – are inhaled by a person who is sensitive to them, hay fever can arise.

Unlike pollen, which has a particular season, moulds are present all the year round in many parts of the world. Their numbers are mainly governed by weather conditions such as rain, wind and temperature. For example, after a spring thaw outdoor moulds begin to flourish, sending ever greater numbers of spores into the air by the warmest days of summer. In climates that are consistently warm, moulds are in evidence throughout the whole year.

Humidity allows mould to propagate and produce spores, and is therefore its greatest ally. Spending time in a damp environment such as a garage or basement can bring on typical allergy symptoms – sneezing, a streaming nose, watering eyes and so on. It is recommended, therefore, that a susceptible person try to remain in places with low humidity (less than 40 per cent).

The amount of mould in the air is measured daily by a variety of methods and the number of grains per cubic metre of air is reported on some websites, along with the daily pollen count. (See Useful addresses at the back of this book for details of a website that gives these counts.)

Outdoor and indoor moulds

Outdoor mould is likely to grow in the following places:

- compost heaps with dead leaves and rotting vegetables
- outbuildings

17

- rotting wood piles
- hay and grain fields
- soil.

Indoor moulds – often referred to as mildew – can give rise to year-round symptoms in a susceptible person. The spores are too minuscule to be seen by the naked eye and particularly thrive in places where air does not circulate freely, such as attics and basements, where there are high levels of humidity, and in places where food is stored, prepared and disposed of. The following are possible areas that attract mould:

- potted plants
- leaky attics
- bathroom shower curtains and rubber non-slip mats
- damp towels and clothing
- pet litter
- around window frames
- rubbish bins
- old mattresses
- leaky pipes and taps
- foam rubber pillows
- refrigerator drip trays and rubber door gaskets
- other food storage areas
- pages of old books (the musty smell is a good indicator that a book is mouldy)
- damp areas of a poorly ventilated room
- damp cellars or basements
- poorly ventilated wardrobes
- over-stuffed furniture
- carpets
- old peeling wallpaper and paint.

Diagnosing an allergy to mould

As medical tests for diagnosing mould allergy are notoriously unreliable, the best way to determine whether or not it is causing you a problem is to avoid contact with moulds of any kind.

Moulds can only survive if they are exposed to moisture in the air; therefore they don't exist in very dry climates. Nor do they flourish at the seaside – moulds don't exist in our seas and oceans, and the prevailing winds blow inland any moulds present in seaside towns.

If you have hay fever symptoms that don't go away when the pollen season ends, it is quite possible that an allergy to mould is your problem. In fact, an allergy to mould is often the reason for year-round hay fever symptoms – perennial hay fever. The best way for you to determine whether or not you have a mould allergy is to go on holiday! The dry climates of places such as southern Spain, the Algarve, the Greek islands or, better still, the Canary Islands would be beneficial environments. Or you may already have found that taking a holiday at the seaside gave you relief from your symptoms. Perhaps you attributed the benefit to fresh air, exercise and a break from stress when, in fact, the improvement was more likely the result of spending time in a mould-free environment.

If mould is indeed an allergen for you, it is important that you keep your particular environment as free from it as possible.

Avoiding mould

Here are some other suggestions for reducing and even eliminating mould in your home, thus creating an allergen-free environment:

- When in the bathroom, open the window or turn on the extractor fan.
- If there are damp areas from water leaks (such areas encourage the growth of mould), it's well worth tackling the problem or asking a plumber to do so for you.
- If you have no choice but to spend time in an area with high humidity, consider purchasing a dehumidifier.
- Think seriously about purchasing an air filter such as the HEPA filter (high efficiency particulate air filter), which can eliminate 99.97 per cent of airborne particles, including fungal spores. There are now a wide variety of such filters available that cut down on spores. Check that the filter you are buying carries some indication that it filters airborne allergens, such as the HEPA label.
- Use an electrostatic filter to minimize the number of airborne contaminants in your home. Electrostatic filters are usually very successful, removing up to 90 per cent of spores.
- As indoor mould is easy detectable to the human eye and nose – it usually appears as a dark greenish furry growth and, in larger areas, smells like mildew – it's always possible to tackle it directly. Use household cleaning products and some elbow grease, or, for more stubborn mould, detergents that are specifically aimed at destroying mould.

Interestingly, ozone generators have been proven successfully to decrease the number of airborne fungal spores. However, it is not yet certain whether they are safe and easy enough to use in the long term. Because more and more people are displaying an allergy to mould, there is a great deal of research under way in this area.

3

Related conditions

Hay fever can be a trial to live with, but in itself is never life-threatening. However, if the symptoms are not controlled, it can lead to complications such as sinus or ear infections. Furthermore, hay fever frequently coexists with other conditions, which often pose more of a problem. Although the most common conditions to coexist with hay fever are eczema and asthma (as discussed later in this chapter), some people are beset with a whole range of allergies and may find it difficult to pinpoint what exactly is causing their symptoms on a particular day. Owing to their chemical make-up, some substances are more allergenic than others.

Possible complications of hay fever

This section discusses the conditions that can arise as a result of hay fever.

Sinus infection

When severe hay fever is not controlled quickly enough, a bacterial infection can result from the inflammation in the nasal and sinus mucous membranes (the tissues that line the nasal and sinus passages). Sinus infections usually require a combination of prescription treatments, including antibiotics and a medication to reduce the congestion. You can also help yourself by employing the following measures:

- Keep a kettle boiling in an enclosed space and breathe in the hot, moist air.
- Apply a hot pack to the areas around the sinuses – gel packs that you can heat up in hot water are available from many chemists. Don't allow the pack to get too hot – it should be bearable.

People with allergies are more likely to develop sinusitis than any other group.

Ear infection

A condition known as *otitis media* – the medical term for a particular type of ear infection – can occur in the space behind the eardrum (the middle ear), causing ear pain and a 'plugged' sensation in the ears. The condition arises due to a series of events which begins with throat inflammation restricting the opening of the Eustachian tube. The Eustachian tube is a narrow passage that leads from the back of the throat to the cavity of the middle ear. It enables pressure on each side of the eardrum to be equalized to enable normal hearing. When the Eustachian tube suffers partial blockage, air is prevented from travelling up it and a slight vacuum in the middle ear results. The vacuum draws fluid from the tissues into the middle ear, causing temporary hearing loss. The fluid is liable to infection in the form of otitis media.

Approximately 80 per cent of otitis media cases clear up within three days, during which time you can use over-the-counter painkillers such as paracetamol or ibuprofen to control the symptoms. If the pain is severe, or getting worse after three days, don't hesitate to visit your doctor, who will prescribe a course of antibiotics. A child under the age of 16 with otitis media should always be seen by a doctor, not simply given over-the-counter medication.

Recurrent bouts of otitis media can eventually lead to hearing loss. However, this can normally be prevented by the use of antibiotic medication.

Rebound nasal congestion

When a decongestant spray is used for more than a few days, the result, ironically, can be increased nose blockage rather than the reverse. Continued use of the spray may then cause chronic inflammation in the delicate mucous membranes – a condition known as *rhinitis medicamentosa* – which makes it difficult to breathe through your nose at all. If you get into this situation, stop using the spray immediately; you will have to put up with a severely blocked nose until such time as you return to the state you were in before you started using the spray.

To be safe, never use a decongestant spray for more than three days.

Nosebleeds

A small number of people with hay fever experience nosebleeds. Fortunately, this is usually a passing problem, occurring on and off over a few weeks. If the bleeds are persistent and really bother you, ask to be referred to an ear, nose and throat specialist at your local hospital. Inflammation may have caused some of the delicate blood vessels in your nose to become particularly fragile and the specialist may offer to remove them by means of cauterization.

This is a minor surgical procedure. If you have just undergone cauterization and you use a nasal spray to deliver medication, avoid damaging the affected nasal membranes by making sure you don't push the nozzle of the applicator against the area. If you are in any doubt, it is probably best to avoid using the spray for two to three weeks after surgery. Your specialist will be able to advise you about this.

Facial changes

Inflammation and congestion in the mucous membranes of the nose and sinuses can give rise to facial swelling, nose redness and puffy eyes. In children with hay fever, frequent wiping can cause a crease across the top of the nose.

Possible accompanying conditions

The conditions associated with hay fever, as described in this section, are essentially inflammatory disorders of the tissues that separate interior regions of the body from the outside world – for example, the skin and the linings of the upper respiratory tract (known as mucous membranes).

Eczema

Having hay fever puts a person at risk of developing eczema, and vice versa. The medical term for eczema is *atopic dermatitis* and is used to describe patches of very itchy, inflamed skin with swelling, redness, weeping, cracking, crusting, scaling and a propensity towards infection. The itching is often all-consuming in eczema, and the subsequent scratching and rubbing unfortunately worsens the skin inflammation and other symptoms. As a result, an 'itch–scratch' cycle results, with the itch demanding to be scratched which in turn worsens the itch. Obviously, trying to stop a small child from scratching an itch is virtually impossible, and even adults with an iron will are likely to scratch in their sleep when conscious control disappears.

There are several different types of eczema; it can develop in infancy or appear later in life, and there are flare-up periods followed by remissions where the skin makes a partial recovery or clears totally. In many people, although their skin may remain dry and easily irritated, remission is permanent as they reach adulthood. In others, environmental factors such as the use of certain detergents or even skincare products continue to provoke a full flare-up. Emotional factors such as stress can also make eczema worse. It cannot *cause* eczema, however.

Eczema is an atopic disease, meaning that it belongs to a group of diseases that run in families and are often present at the same time. For instance, an individual prone to both eczema and asthma may find that during an eczema flare-up an asthma attack is experienced too. Eczema affects males and females equally, with approximately 90 per cent of sufferers developing the condition before the age of five. Living in an urban area with higher levels of car exhaust fumes and industrial pollutants appears to increase the risk of developing the condition.

Isolating and avoiding the triggering factor is not always easy. Obvious irritants can be avoided, but the mainstay of eczema management is the regular use of good skin-softening preparations such as aqueous cream and, where necessary, steroid creams such as hydrocortisone (brand name Hc45). Such products block incoming allergens by making a temporary artificial barrier on the skin. They are therefore able to interrupt the cycle of barrier breakdown, attempted repair and further breakdown. Subsequently, the immune system should calm down and cell growth decelerate.

Unfortunately, some of the barrier creams used can cause undesired side effects such as dermatitis, pustules, broken blood vessels and loss of skin colour. Your doctor will, therefore, need to monitor your progress very carefully.

Because many children with eczema go on to develop the more serious asthma, they may also be treated with medications that suppress the immune system and so prevent asthma from arising – examples are ciclosporin (also spelt cyclosporine) (brand name USAN) and azathioprine (brand name Imuran). These medications can also cause undesirable side effects, however, such as adverse reactions with other medications, diarrhoea, vomiting, fever and convulsions.

Psoriasis

Psoriasis, also a very itchy condition, is believed to arise in the same way as eczema – that is, due to a breakdown in the skin barrier which allows allergens to pass through, stimulate the immune system to produce extra skin cells and create the cycle of barrier breakdown. Psoriasis is often present with hay fever and eczema, indicating that it, too, may have a genetic factor. Indeed, studies have shown that the condition arises in as many as 50 per cent of siblings when one parent is affected. Not everyone with psoriasis has a family history of the disorder, however.

Psoriasis can arise at any age, and both sexes stand an equal chance of developing it. The condition can occur in a susceptible person when they experience a particular trigger; such triggers may include the following:

- Psoriasis can appear at the site of a trauma – following a skin scrape, scratch or cut (such as a surgical wound), or at areas of sunburn.
- Emotional stress can cause an acceleration of the condition.
- Psoriasis is a risk factor for certain medications such as the mood-stabilizing drug lithium (brand name Eskalith) and several of the anti-malarial drugs.
- It can occur during a systemic infection – where the whole body is affected – such as influenza.

It is interesting to note that in people with psoriasis, there is a substantially lower incidence of the two main types of eczema: allergic contact dermatitis and atopic dermatitis. This strongly suggests that the immune system disturbances evident in psoriasis are different from those evident in the two types of eczema. When the genetic make-up of eczema and psoriasis are eventually discovered, we will have a better understanding of the more serious related disorders such as asthma.

Psoriasis differs visually from eczema in that there are *lesions* (also referred to as *plaques*) with well-defined edges and silvery scales that easily flake off. Beneath the scales, the skin appears shiny and red. This tends to be a lifelong condition and is characterized by bouts of flaring and clearing. A remission (where the skin is clear) may last for several months or even years.

If you have psoriasis, your dermatologist will strongly advise that you follow a daily hygiene routine to limit the possibility of bacteria invading the area of skin damage and setting up a secondary infection. Increased reddening and greater heat in the affected area and/or the presence of pus are indicators of a secondary infection. These are generally accompanied by light-headedness, fever and a general feeling of being unwell. As a skin abrasion can trigger the formation of further lesions, it is also recommended that you try hard not to scratch the area. Rubbing, picking or scrubbing the lesion should also be avoided.

In winter, humidity levels are generally lower than at other times of the year, particularly in homes with central heating. As a result the skin of a person with psoriasis may become drier and itchier. The best way to manage the condition is to use plenty of moisturizing creams, especially during the winter, paying particular attention to the areas affected by psoriasis. For the best results, the cream or ointment should be applied while the skin is still damp after washing or bathing. It is also important to pat your skin dry after bathing rather than rubbing with a towel. Many people have flare-ups of psoriasis lesions between their toes and they should, at all costs, avoid pulling a towel to and fro between their toes.

Your doctor will probably prescribe certain skin-softening preparations, as well as a steroid cream. In more severe cases, medication may also be prescribed, such as methotrexate (brand name Rheumatrex) and ciclosporin (brand name USAN).

Asthma

Most people who suffer from asthma also have other allergies, which may include hay fever. Asthma affects people of all ages, but often develops in childhood. Boys are more likely to have asthma than girls, but in adulthood, more women are likely to be affected than men.

In brief, asthma is a chronic disease in which a person's airways become inflamed and are therefore sensitive to certain substances, known as irritants or allergens (see pages 10–11 for a description of an allergic reaction). The allergic reaction in asthma causes the airways to become narrower, allowing less air through to the lungs. Extra mucus is also produced, and these two things together make breathing difficult, causing wheezing, coughing and chest tightness.

Asthma attacks vary a great deal in intensity. If very severe, the airways can actually close so that insufficient oxygen reaches the lungs and other vital organs. This situation constitutes a medical emergency, as anaphylactic shock (see page 45) and even death can result – though in very rare cases. If you have asthma, your doctor will prescribe medication such as salbutamol (brand name Ventolin) or montelukast (brand name Singulair) which it is important that you keep with you wherever you go. Recognizing and avoiding your particular triggers can make a vast difference. The same allergenic substances as in hay fever can trigger attacks, such as pollen, mould spores, dung from house dust mites and animal dander.

The following can also trigger an asthma attack:

- stress
- environmental pollutants

- strongly perfumed household products
- tobacco smoke
- changes in weather
- cold air
- strong-smelling paints
- extremes of emotional expression, such as laughing and crying.

People with asthma often find that their wheezing and breathlessness worsen during a hay fever episode. Indeed, some people experience asthma symptoms only in the course of the hay fever season. Researchers have suggested that an exacerbation of any other allergy can either cause or worsen an asthma attack.

If you think that you might have symptoms of asthma and have not yet seen your doctor, you should do so as soon as possible. Tests will help to diagnose the condition, after which you will be offered the appropriate treatment.

Oral allergy syndrome

In addition to the allergens already mentioned – pollen, mould, dust, feathers, animal dander, chemicals and environmental pollutants – edible items can also provoke a reaction in susceptible people. This is a condition known as oral allergy syndrome (OAS), also sometimes referred to as the pollen-food allergy syndrome. The symptoms arising are largely restricted to the mouth and throat. Eating fruit, for example, has been reported to result in itching of the mouth and throat, mouth ulcers, swelling of the lips and/or tongue, hoarseness and a need for compulsive throat clearing. When the oral allergen is cooked or canned, the reaction doesn't appear to occur.

Foods of the *compositae* group – the aster family of plants – such as nuts, celery, lettuce, artichoke, chicory, sunflower and safflower can give rise to acute allergic reactions with serious symptoms such as swollen throat and vocal cords, bronchial asthma, urticaria (nettle rash) and sometimes even anaphylactic shock.

Having an allergy to a specific type of pollen can make you susceptible to developing an allergy to a particular food or foods. Indeed, the following observations have been made:

- People who react to silver birch pollen (prevalent in Europe and Asia) often develop an oral allergy to apples, cherries, peaches, carrots, celery, walnuts, peanuts and hazelnuts.

- People who are allergic to grass pollen (dominant in many areas of the world) tend to develop an oral allergy to melon, watermelon and tomatoes.
- People who are allergic to mugwort (prevalent in Europe, Asia and Africa) often develop an allergy to apple, carrot and celery.
- People who react to ragweed (prevalent in North America) tend to develop an allergy to honey, bananas and melon.

In the same way, people who are allergic to latex – latex gloves, for example – are prone to developing allergies to bananas, kiwi fruit, avocado and chestnut.

In a study of 1,129 adults with hay fever and/or bronchial asthma, a substantial 24 per cent experienced allergy symptoms on eating or even handling certain foods – hazelnut, shellfish and apple being the worst culprits.[3] Interestingly, the same researchers also discovered a link between an allergy to birch tree pollen and food sensitivity to apple, cherry, nuts, peach, carrot, plum and new potato. In allergy tests, it was seen that those with the severest allergy to birch pollen were sensitive to a wider array of foods. In addition, the study found a correlation between intolerance to acetylsalicylic acid (a food additive) and sensitivity to foods such as nuts, strawberries, chocolate, almonds, rosehips, green pepper, milk, cabbage and eggs. Considering the large amounts of food additives consumed in the average Western diet, it is no wonder that so many people become sensitive to certain foods. (See pages 83–7 for a discussion of the foods to avoid in hay fever.)

It might seem surprising that even a natural food such as honey can trigger a strong allergic reaction in people with hay fever, as research has shown. In further tests, this was explained by the large concentration of sunflower pollen (23.6 per cent) found in the honey, and it was this that was responsible for provoking the reaction.[4] Allergic reactions from other natural foods such as sunflower and safflower – from which many oils on our supermarket shelves are produced – are also thought to be caused by pollen.

A food elimination programme

Discovering whether you are sensitive to a particular type of food can be very difficult; tests are available, but each can be criticized if one deliberately sets out to do so. The only certain way to prove the case is via a food elimination programme. As this requires the elimination of one food at a time, then waiting to assess your body's response, it would take many months to find your sensitivities. For this reason, attending an allergy clinic is advisable.

Initial withdrawal reaction

If you already suspect, however, that certain foods are causing you problems, a food elimination programme can be a good idea. Withdraw one food at a time from your diet for one month. Assuming that the food you eliminate is indeed a problem, there is often an initial withdrawal reaction – fatigue, headaches, twitching and irritability are normal, and can persist for up to 15 days. Drinking around five pints of water each day can help to reduce these symptoms. This can also aid detoxification and help to flush any residual offending foods through the digestive system.

Halfway through the elimination programme you may find that you become hypersensitive to the culprit food and that eating it unwittingly can cause a severe reaction. Dining out during this period may be inadvisable, as you never know exactly what ingredients have been used. If you are eating out, ask the chef, not the waiter, if you are at all uncertain of the ingredients.

A pleasing symptom of food elimination can be weight loss, if you were overweight. The reason for this is that many people with food sensitivities have an excess of fluid distributed throughout their bodies. When they eliminate certain suspect foods, this fluid quickly drains away.

While you are following a food elimination programme, make sure that you continue to eat enough staple foods such as bread, cereals, rice, pasta, fruit (see Chapter 7) and vegetables. Cutting down too much can lead to nutritional deficiencies. If you need to eliminate some staple foods from your diet, ensure that you take a multivitamin and mineral supplement to prevent any possible deficiencies.

Reintroduction of excluded foods

Towards the end of the month you may be feeling better than you have for a long time. The sense of well-being can be so great that you won't want to bother to reintroduce the excluded foods. But if you do wish to reintroduce them, the following procedure is suggested:

- *Day 1*: In the morning, reintroduce a small amount of an eliminated food (not a full-sized portion). Do the same later in the day and take note of any symptoms.
- *Day 2*: If you fail to experience symptoms, repeat the exercise. Once again, take note of any symptoms. If you get through the second day, this is really good news. Now wait two more days before you can safely reintroduce this food into your diet on a fairly regular basis.

Repeat this four-day reintroduction procedure with each food eliminated. Any reintroduction side effect should have occurred within this period. Unfortunately, you may find that some foods will always cause an adverse reaction, so it is wise to withdraw them from your diet completely. In the meantime, continue to eat sensibly. Try not to indulge too much in the foods that previously caused problems. And remember, if in doubt, leave it out!

See Chapter 7 for a nutritional approach to treating hay fever.

4

The causes of hay fever

The number of hay fever cases has been rising steadily over the last few decades and continues to do so. There have been reports of a fourfold increase in the number of hay fever patients consulting their doctors, and it has been argued that this is partly because people are becoming more health-aware and actively seeking answers to their problems. This is undoubtedly true, but should not screen the fact that there has been a real and dramatic increase in the number of people with hay fever, especially in Western societies.

The reasons for the increase are hotly debated and I imagine will continue to be so for some time. The explanations that have thus far been put forward are discussed in this chapter.

Oilseed rape

It has been suggested that the rise in hay fever cases is in some part due to a great increase in the cultivation of oilseed rape, an annual plant of the mustard family. Oilseed rape, which is used in the manufacture of margarine and cooking oils, is the new cash crop, producing masses of yellow flowers and a distinctive smell. Indeed, the bright yellow fields are widely seen in our countryside and are set to cover yet more cultivated land.

Although some people blame their hay fever symptoms on the pollen from oilseed rape, research has shown that scarcely 4 per cent are allergic to it – and only in the month of May. However, people who live close to oilseed rape fields often complain of a runny nose, watering eyes and throat irritation – which are symptoms of hay fever. Allergy experts state, however, that this reaction cannot be classified as an allergy as it is not actually triggered by the pollen from oilseed rape. They explain that the cold-like symptoms are more likely to be caused by the potent (but organic) chemicals produced by the crop – these give rise to the strong smell. Such chemicals, therefore, are classed as 'irritants' and cause sensitivity rather than an allergic reaction.

The decline of areas of grassland

Pollen from grass is actually the main irritant for the majority of people with hay fever – it is also a true allergen – yet areas of grassland in the UK and other countries are now significantly reduced. As a result, pollen counts have actually declined since the early 1960s. So the question is: why, even when pollen counts are falling, does hay fever continue to gain momentum, with more and more people experiencing symptoms each year?

Adrenal exhaustion

Many allergy experts believe that the root cause of allergic disease, including hay fever, is adrenal exhaustion. The adrenal glands sit on top of the kidneys; their core produces vital adrenalin which 'fires' the heart. However, excessive amounts of mental, physical and/or emotional stress make them pump more adrenalin than necessary; this overworking is obviously very draining for them and can cause them to weaken and malfunction. This is why stress control is so important in allergy conditions such as hay fever. (See pages 73–5 for a relaxation programme which helps to counter stress.)

An important function of the outer regions of the adrenal glands – the cortex – is the production of about 50 hormones and other substances which play key roles in virtually every bodily function. It makes sense, then, to say that adrenal exhaustion leads to problems in many areas. One of the hormones produced by these glands is cortisone, which works with others to mediate the body's inflammatory response. When the adrenal cortex is weakened, however, a variety of inflammatory problems can occur, including asthma, hay fever and eczema.

Each of the adrenal hormones requires vitamin C to maintain their function, and for this reason that particular vitamin is vital for controlling hay fever symptoms (see Chapter 7 for more information on vitamin C). It also appears that the adrenal cortex is very sensitive to blood sugar levels, and the intake of large amounts of refined carbohydrates such as those in biscuits, some breads and pasta, cakes, sweets and pastries is the deep-rooted cause of many allergies. However, taking cortisone by mouth has been found to actually weaken the adrenal glands over time, and so experts believe that the optimum means of strengthening and supporting the adrenal glands is through a nutritional programme, including nutritional supplements, to rebuild and rebalance the adrenal cortex. See Chapter 7 for a nutritional approach to hay fever, which is believed to tackle the root cause of the condition. When the adrenal glands are functioning more efficiently, virtually every bodily system improves. Qualified nutritionists now offer a test to determine adrenal exhaustion.

If you are experiencing a situation that is particularly stressful or have unresolved emotional issues, it is advisable to see a skilled counsellor. Stress depletes levels of vitamin C in the body.

Exposure to pollutants

The last 50 years have seen scientific advances that could barely have been guessed at in our grandparents' day. Vaccinations, medications and procedures have been developed which literally save lives, and synthetic chemicals that may have caused industry to boom and made housework and personal care so much easier. It is a sad fact, however, that these marvellous advances are slowly weakening our immune systems and draining our adrenal glands, for we ingest a small amount of the toxins they emit every day. Indeed, they are entering our bodies all the time through our skin, nasal passages and digestive tracts.

Many allergy experts and environmentalists are of the opinion that the increase in pollution levels in Western societies is one reason for the sharp rise in hay fever cases. There is certainly far more pollution from such things as industry, tobacco smoke and car exhaust fumes, and the airways of susceptible individuals can become sensitive to repeated exposure. This is the reason that some car mechanics become sensitive to petrol fumes, some painters to paint, some printers to ink, and so on.

It is said that a person's potential for developing allergies depends upon the amount of irritants their body can take before an allergy results. We all vary a great deal in the number of toxins, pollutants and so on that our bodies can tolerate, and that variation appears to be closely linked, in the first place, to the following:

- The ability of our immune systems to determine accurately innocuous substances from potentially harmful ones. An immune system that does not correctly identify certain substances is said to be weakened or 'sensitized'.
- The vitality of our adrenal glands. Healthy adrenal glands produce many important hormones which interact in the body as they should. Exhausted adrenal glands, on the other hand, get confused and produce too little of these hormones, causing interactions that may be damaging to the body.

A person with an already sensitized immune system and exhausted adrenal glands is far more prone to developing allergies than a person with a strong immune system and healthy adrenal glands.

So what causes the immune system to become sensitized and the adrenal glands to get exhausted in the first place, you might ask. The answer is often prolonged and repeated exposure to irritants. However, not everyone who is exposed on a daily basis to pollen, for example, will develop hay fever, as we know. One or more other factors must also be thrown into the mix, such as:

- having a family member with allergies;
- being raised in an over-sterile environment (as discussed later in this chapter);
- eating a poor diet (nutritional advice is given in Chapter 7);
- being overexposed to antibiotics in childhood (as discussed later in this chapter).

The main environmental pollutants in the West are carbon monoxide, sulphur dioxide, chlorofluorocarbons (CFCs) and nitrogen oxides, all of which are produced by industry and motor vehicles. In addition, minute proteins on pollen grains can be washed off by the rain and stick to toxic particles in the polluted air. These particles can then – because they are so tiny – be drawn right down into the lungs, increasing the chances of an allergic reaction.

Prolonged and repeated chemical exposure

People who work in certain environments – factories, garages, hairdressing salons, chemical plants, and on farms – are exposed to chemicals on a daily basis. They may find that, if they are predisposed in any way to developing allergies, they start being troubled by such things as hives, itching, skin eruptions, runny nose, sneezing, respiratory problems, diarrhoea, tinnitus, cramps and excessive fatigue. In time, the immune system may even begin to react against the chemicals themselves.

Air-conditioning in offices also puts a person at risk of developing allergies, for it continually recycles irritants and pollutants such as tobacco smoke, perfumes, toiletries, moulds, bacteria and viruses around the building. Nor are our homes safe havens from chemicals – far from it in most cases. We tend to use an array of cleaning substances that can lead to allergies in susceptible people. In addition, most of us inadvertently use a staggering amount of chemicals in our personal grooming products and don't think to read the list of ingredients on the packet or can. Fortunately, there is an increasing range of more natural products which are becoming widely available.

Indoor air contaminants

Indoor air contaminants include building materials, paints, varnish, glues, plastics, carpeting, new furnishings, insecticides, disinfectants, detergents, dyes, and gas leakage from stoves and heaters. Personal care products such as deodorants, skin lotions, cosmetics, perfumes, shower gels, hair shampoo and conditioners can also provoke adverse reactions in sensitive individuals. It is well worth looking for biologically friendly products that won't act as irritants. These can be found in some high street chemists or obtained from specialist manufacturers and suppliers of nutritional supplements. Don't take the words 'natural' and 'pure' on labels as gospel – there is no onus on manufacturers to stick to the literal truth of these words.

Outdoor air contaminants

Outdoor air contaminants include industrial fumes, traffic exhaust fumes, smog, crop-spraying and the paving and resurfacing of roads. Synthetic drugs – that is, those derived from petroleum – are a common source of sensitivity, too. The colourings and flavourings in medications and foods can also cause problems.

The only answer to all this is to reduce your exposure to all irritants, including chemicals. If this means changing your job, it's certainly a big deal – but it's going to be better than weakening your bodily systems even further and risking an increasingly greater allergic response. In addition, following the diet recommended in Chapter 7, as well as taking the recommended nutritional supplements (also discussed in Chapter 7), may reduce your sensitivity to chemicals.

Organophosphates

One of the most common chemical sensitivities is to organophosphates (OPs), which are widely used in farming throughout the Western world. OPs are highly toxic chemicals that are used as a matter of course for pest control in crop production and animal husbandry. They are also used in home pesticides such as fly sprays. Originally developed to attack the central nervous system in warfare, in order to kill, they can adversely affect every bodily system and are believed to be implicated in the onset of allergies. OPs are never used in organic farming, however.

Detox your body of OPs by avoiding exposure to pesticides, following an organic diet, and taking vitamin and mineral supplements. Vitamins A, C, E and B12, and magnesium and selenium are particularly effective.

Heavy metals

Besides chemicals, our bodies are absorbing small quantities of heavy metals every day. Hair mineral analysis, which can be undertaken through a qualified nutritionist, can indicate high levels of certain minerals. The worst culprits are as follows:

- *Aluminium* – Because high levels of aluminium can cause severe damage to several of the body's systems, it is best avoided. Sources of aluminium poisoning are some underarm deodorants, aluminium cookware, aluminium foil and foil containers. Surprisingly, this metal can also be found in coffee, bleached white flour and some antacid medications.
- *Mercury* – Individuals with amalgam tooth fillings are ingesting minute amounts of mercury vapour every day, and mercury is the second most toxic heavy metal in the world. The leaked mercury vapour can gradually weaken the immune system, making it hypersensitive to irritants. Synthetic white fillings are a safe alternative.
- *Cadmium* – High carbohydrate consumption is now thought to be linked with high cadmium levels in the body. Cigarette-smoking is another cause of cadmium build-up, cadmium being mainly absorbed through the lungs. This metal is known to be damaging to the kidneys and respiratory system. It can, however, be gradually removed by following a healthy, organic diet such as that discussed in Chapter 7.

An over-sterile environment

In the mid-1990s, David Strachan, now professor of epidemiology at St George's Hospital in London, put forward the hypothesis that our increasingly sterile environments are exposing young people to fewer infections as they grow, which prevents their immune systems from maturing. It is certainly true that, nowadays, many of us try to keep our homes free of viruses and bacteria, using disinfectant sprays, creams and wipes to stop infections occurring. We are seemingly too zealous in our efforts to fight the germs, however, for not only do we keep infections at bay, we are inadvertently allowing underdeveloped immune systems – usually those of our children – to mistakenly identify pollen and certain other innocuous substances as foreign invaders.

Professor Strachan also observed that first-born children are more likely to develop hay fever and asthma than their younger siblings. The reason that younger siblings are more robust, he suggested, was that as well as infections in the home environment, they have to contend with infections brought home by older siblings. Their immune systems, therefore, have more to work with, which allows them to become more efficient. I would add that parents are more likely to keep the germs at bay when there is only one child. When other children come along, parents generally have less time to spend on cleaning compared with other demands on their attention. Professor Strachan's hypothesis has, in recent years, been confirmed by several research studies.

Research has also indicated that children who attend pre-school day nurseries from an early age are less likely to succumb to allergies – including hay fever and asthma – than children who are kept at home until they are three, four or five years old.

Antibiotics

There has been a great deal of scientific debate in recent years into whether children who take antibiotics are at greater risk of developing allergies than those who don't. Despite several studies into a possible link between antibiotics and allergy development, we don't yet have a definitive answer.

A number of study reports have suggested that allergies are in fact more likely to develop in people who took antibiotics as young children, whereas others indicate that this is not the case. It would appear, however, that studies showing a positive correlation between antibiotics and allergies are generally flawed. For instance, in one study, consumption of antibiotics in the first five years of life showed a definite link between the development of asthma and other allergies.[5] It was believed, though, that the link was the result of medications prescribed for respiratory disorders – indeed, the authors of the study concluded that such respiratory system disorders must have eventually led to the development of further respiratory problems.

Studies that attempt to show an association between antibiotic use and the development of allergies in children are always at risk of being clouded by unrecognized asthma. That is, coughs, wheezes and such may be treated by antibiotic medication when the child is, in fact, displaying early symptoms of asthma. Studies which have focused instead on people with symptoms unrelated to asthma are therefore believed to give a clearer picture of the real situation. One such study has shown a link, but one that was not of statistical significance.[6] Moreover, this study looked back at the first 30 years of life of its subjects, failing to take into account the fact that asthma has greatly increased in prevalence over that time. The subjects in the study had been issued an average of three antibiotics prescriptions a year for five years. A more recent study into the average usage of prescription antibiotics indicated that the real average may be as high as ten prescriptions a year.[7]

Probiotics

Recent studies have focused on probiotics in relation to allergic disease. Probiotics are dietary supplements that contain active cultures of beneficial bacteria (yeast). They are believed to help healthy intestinal flora re-establish themselves after a course of antibiotics has been taken. Interestingly, when given to subjects in a number of controlled trials, they appeared to lower the risk of allergic disease. This strongly suggests that antibiotics raise the risk. Nutritionists state, therefore, that keeping the intestinal flora healthy is a great defence against allergic diseases such as asthma, eczema and hay fever.

Probiotic supplements usually contain healthy bacteria called *acidophilus* (see page 70). It is rather like liquid yogurt and pleasant to the taste buds. Actimel and Yakult are respected probiotic brand names and are available from most supermarkets. Other foodstuffs also contain probiotics, such as certain yogurts. A pregnant woman can take probiotics to protect her unborn child, and a breastfeeding mother can take probiotics to protect her baby.

Help for parents

If you are reluctant for your child to take antibiotics, what should you do if your doctor recommends that a course is needed? My best advice is as follows:

- As there are often medical alternatives to antibiotics, ask your doctor if another safe treatment for your child's infection can be prescribed.
- Ask your doctor to recommend a good non-drug-oriented treatment. Whether or not your doctor agrees to let you try another approach will depend on the severity of your child's particular infection, and the doctor's own treatment beliefs and leanings.

- If it is vital that your child take a course of antibiotics, ask your doctor if it is possible to be prescribed the most appropriate narrow-spectrum choice. Antibiotics are available that can target particular offending bacteria. Broad-spectrum antibiotics tend to kill beneficial intestinal flora (beneficial bacteria) as well as killing the culprit bacteria.
- When your child has finished a course of antibiotics, a probiotic supplement is recommended, such as acidophilus, which will help rebalance the intestinal bacteria. If you need further information on this, ask your pharmacist.

An inherited tendency

Many people are genetically programmed to be susceptible to allergies. In other words, they are born with an inherited tendency to become allergic to certain substances – particularly substances with which they come into repeated contact. This means that you and your siblings are more likely to develop hay fever (and other allergies) if one of your parents have (or had) hay fever or other allergic conditions such as eczema, asthma, urticaria and true food allergies.

When a person with a genetic tendency to developing allergies comes in contact with other causative factors such as environmental toxins, the likelihood of their developing one or more allergies is increased.

Holistic versus conventional treatment

Since conventional medicines – with the exception of immunotherapy (see Chapter 5 for information about conventional medications) – can only offer palliative help, many people with allergies choose to try a holistic approach. This involves treating oneself as a whole – mind, body and soul – in an effort to tackle the underlying problems.

In brief, the holistic approach to treating hay fever involves the following:

- supporting exhausted adrenal glands so their hormone production returns to normal;
- providing appropriate nutritional support to nourish cells and improve all areas;
- using a combination of vitamin and mineral supplementation, together with herbal support and other natural remedies, to strengthen the immune system and reduce its hypersensitivity;

- reducing stress and learning how to relax;
- learning how to feel good about yourself.

Whether you choose to try conventional treatments, holistic therapy or a combination of both, the rest of this book attempts to inform you about all the treatments and therapies currently available so you can make your own choices.

5

The medical help available

You may not like to bother your doctor with symptoms as common-place as sneezing, a runny nose and watery eyes – but if you are unable to control such symptoms, medical help should really be sought. Any health problem that you are unable successfully to self-treat, whether or not it appears trivial, should be mentioned to your doctor. There may be a course of available treatment that, when followed, makes a great deal of difference to your life. Even when you suspect that no treatment is currently available – I'm talking about other conditions besides hay fever here – your doctor should be informed and the symptoms duly noted on your records. A treatment may become avail-able at a later date, or the problem may be found to tie in with later symptoms to form a complete picture and allow a diagnosis.

Of course, hay fever is sometimes nothing more than a minor in-convenience that can be controlled by reducing exposure to the allergen(s) responsible. It is when symptoms actively interfere with your normal routine at work, at home and during leisure activities that you should go to your doctor.

If your hay fever is accompanied by asthma, or you are not sure that your particular allergens are pollen and mould, you should definitely seek medical advice.

Making the diagnosis

Where hay fever is concerned, your doctor is likely to be able to diag-nose the allergy from a description of your symptoms. The time of day at which your symptoms are worst is an important factor, but always try to give your doctor a complete and accurate picture – hay fever symptoms increase at a certain time of the day in some people depend-ing upon their particular allergen(s). These are questions your doctor is likely to ask:

- During the course of a day, when exactly are your symptoms at their worst?

41

- During the course of a day, when exactly do your symptoms improve, if at all?
- At what time of the year are your symptoms at their worst?
- Can you anticipate when your symptoms are about to start? If so, what are the signs?
- Do any of your family members suffer from allergies?
- Are your symptoms worse when you are around pets?
- Have you noticed whether other substances – such as household cleaning products – make your symptoms worse? If so, what are the substances in question?

If the diagnosis is not obvious, skin or blood tests may be taken in order to determine your particular allergy. People who have year-round symptoms – perennial hay fever – may be found to be allergic not only to pollen but to mould spores, the dung from house dust mites, fur from pets, feathers in duck down pillows and so on.

Currently, there are insufficient allergy specialists in the UK to deal with what has become a considerable problem, and few GPs are trained to treat allergies. However, the allergy specialists we do have are trained to a high standard. Their training programme usually extends to several years of education, and an evaluation process which includes an examination to demonstrate their knowledge, skills and expertise in patient care. Therefore, if your doctor doesn't appear to be too interested in your problem, it's highly recommended that you ask for a referral to an allergy specialist, referred to as an *allergist*.

If you are being treated at your local surgery, your doctor will check your medical history and ask if you are aware of any other allergies. Your answer will indicate whether or not you are an allergy-prone individual and therefore more likely to have hay fever; it will also help your doctor to prescribe a safe treatment – some people who are prone to allergies react adversely to certain medication.

Treatment

The main aim of hay fever treatment is to allow you to lead a more normal life. It is not essential that treatment should eradicate every last symptom – a definite reduction of symptoms will allow you to do the things you want to do and get enjoyment from them. Hay fever medications are available both on prescription and over-the-counter (without the need for a prescription), depending upon their individual strength and potency.

If you are unhappy with the results of the first treatment you are offered or prescribed, ask your doctor or allergy specialist if you can try something else. A combination of treatments may work best for you, but it may take trial and error, as well as a deal of perseverance, to find the optimum combination.

The following are the main treatments available for hay fever:

- *Antihistamines* – Medications containing antihistamine counter the effects of the chemicals released naturally in the body during an allergic reaction. As a result, sneezing, a runny nose, an itchy throat and watering eyes are relieved.
- *Anti-allergy agents* – These are likely to be composed of a chemical called sodium cromoglicate, which is capable of halting the production of histamine and so can prevent an allergic reaction.
- *Decongestants* – A short, sharp dose of this medication can help to unblock any nasal congestion. Long-term use is not recommended as it can worsen the situation.
- *Steroidal nasal sprays* – These have an anti-inflammatory effect which decreases swelling in the eyes and delicate mucous membranes of the nose.

The above treatments are discussed in more detail later in this chapter. However, the treatment you are offered is likely to depend on the factors mentioned below. If you feel that your lifestyle needs are not being taken into account by your doctor or allergy specialist, be very clear in saying how you need to be able to function better on all levels.

The severity of your symptoms

Severe hay fever may respond best to three or four treatments in combination, whereas milder hay fever will normally respond well to an antihistamine medication alone – perhaps an over-the-counter type – or maybe a nasal spray as well. Very mild hay fever may require no medical intervention and be successfully treated by the employment of self-help measures, as discussed in Chapter 6.

The nature of your worst symptoms

If watering eyes are your worst symptom, you will need the relevant eye drops (as described below in this chapter), whereas if a runny nose is your main problem, an antihistamine medication may be your best option, together with short-term use of a decongestant, if necessary.

The needs of your particular lifestyle

A person who works behind the scenes, in theatre props for example, may not feel as troubled and embarrassed by their symptoms as someone who is very visible to others, such as an actor or a teacher. In the same way, someone who uses their hands for a set length of time, such as a musician during a recital, will find it impossible to play while suffering from a runny nose and watering eyes, whereas those who work alone, say in a home office, will not have quite the same concerns. When your doctor or allergist is considering your treatment regime, your hobbies and any other lifestyle activities should be taken into account just as much as employment factors.

Make it clear how important it is that the very best of treatments should be offered to young people such as those whose symptoms make schoolwork a trial, who are about to take exams, or who have job interviews coming up.

Hay fever and lifestyle are discussed in greater detail in Chapter 9.

Nasal discharge test

If your doctor suspects that hay fever is your problem and your nose is very runny at the time, a drop of the discharge can be taken and examined under a microscope. Immune system cells called *eosinophils* multiply rapidly when the body is fighting off what it sees as an invader; therefore a large number of them clearly indicates the presence of an allergic reaction, that is, hay fever.

Skin prick test

Skin prick testing is the preferred means of determining the presence of specific IgE antibodies (see page 4) and should indicate whether or not allergy treatment is an option for you. The skin prick test – also known as puncture testing, owing to the series of tiny punctures made in the patient's skin – is likely to be carried out in the immunology department of your local hospital and provided by an immunologist with advanced training in the diagnosis and treatment of allergic disease. This type of test is easier to use, faster, more accurate and less expensive than other available methods. Indeed, it is considered the best allergy test currently available.

If you take antihistamines, you will be asked to refrain from taking them for several days prior to the skin prick test being carried out.

On the day of the test, the skin on the inside of your forearm or an area on your back is marked by the immunologist with a special non-allergenic pen or dye, and then a small plastic or metal implement is used to puncture the skin in several places. Into each puncture a tiny amount of a few substances to which you may be allergic is inserted. In some cases, a needle and syringe are used to inject suspected allergens beneath the skin.

Although an individual may be convinced that they have identified their own particular allergic sensitivity, the skin prick test will often prove a different culprit. Therefore, even if you think you know what is causing your problem, it is recommended that you undergo a skin prick test.

People who have a skin condition of any kind will be offered a blood test rather than the skin prick test, as will individuals who have been unable to avoid antihistamine use for several days prior to the test.

The result

After 30 minutes any allergic response will be evident; this will vary from a slight reddening of the skin in a less sensitive person to a swollen, livid-looking weal (commonly known as a 'hive') in a more sensitive person. Any swelling, itching and irritation is likely to be treated and calmed by the application of a soothing cream to the area tested. The immunologist then measures the level of IgE antibodies produced by the body to fight the 'invading' substance. The symbol +/– means that a borderline reaction was provoked; 2+ would describe a moderate reaction, while 4+ would indicate a large reaction.

Obviously, if an extreme reaction has previously occurred, in the form of life-threatening anaphylactic shock – where large quantities of chemicals are released very quickly into the bloodstream causing a sudden drop in blood pressure and difficulty breathing – the substance believed to be responsible will not be introduced into the body and a blood test will be taken instead. Fortunately, hay fever does not provoke such an extreme reaction as anaphylactic shock.

A delayed response

In a small number of people, a delayed response may become apparent up to six hours after the skin prick test, and the redness or weal can persist for up to 72 hours. You will have been given instructions about what to do in the event of such an occurrence. If you experience this type of delayed reaction, don't hesitate to telephone the number you have been given. You may be called back to the hospital, and the immunologist will be able to interpret the reaction and offer an anti-inflammatory cream which you will need to apply regularly until it settles down.

The eyelid test

This is a less common form of skin-testing. The suspected allergen is diluted, and dropped on to the lower eyelid. Any allergic reaction is then noted. This test can be harmful if not carried out correctly, so it should always be done by an allergy specialist and not by the patient.

Blood serum test

The blood test is a useful diagnostic tool; the serum part of it is used to calculate how effective the immune system is in fighting diseases. In seeking evidence of allergies, the aim of the blood test – also known as the 'total IgE level' – is to measure the levels of IgE antibodies present in the person's bloodstream. Various test methods are used to determine the levels of IgE that relate to specific allergenic substances. For instance, the radioallergosorbent test (known as RAST) employs radioactive isotopes to measure IgE levels, and they can also be measured by means of colormetric or fluorometric technology. Basically, the immunologist screening the test is looking for a definitive 'yes' or 'no' as to whether or not an allergic sensitivity to a particular substance is present, and the above tests normally provide this.

Where the result is not conclusive, sensitization to allergens that are commonly inhaled cannot be ruled out. The actual test requires that a few drops of blood are taken from a vein, usually on the inner side of the elbow. Often a cord or tourniquet is fastened quite tightly around the upper arm to prevent blood flow, and this effectively makes the vein more prominent. The tourniquet may feel rather tight, but any discomfort is soon over. The nurse or doctor taking the test will clean the area with spirit, insert the needle into the vein and pull the plunger back to draw blood into the attached syringe. Once the needle is withdrawn a piece of cotton wool is placed over the tiny wound and you will be asked to press down on this. A couple of minutes later, a sticking plaster is placed over the area.

Do tell the nurse or doctor if you suffer from a needle phobia and feel faint at the sight of your own blood. The test can then be carried out while you are lying down to reduce any faintness. If you feel at all faint, don't hesitate to speak up.

Unfortunately, the blood serum test does not always give a positive result, even in the presence of an allergy.

Antihistamine

As the name suggests, antihistamine works to combat the release of histamine – the natural chemical discharged by the body during an allergic reaction which is involved in creating inflammation. This drug is a manufactured chemical that is so similar to natural histamine that the mast cells in the lining of the nose, mouth and eyes (see page 12) are fooled into believing it is real and so accept its presence. However, it is not identical, as it would then provoke the cells to cause allergy symptoms. Therefore, antihistamine effectively blocks many of the body's histamine receptors, preventing them from producing the symptoms of an allergic reaction. Antihistamine is a basic treatment of urticaria (also called hives or nettle rash) as well as hay fever. It used to be employed as a treatment for asthma, too, but now in Western societies there are many more sophisticated asthma medications.

There is a problem with using antihistamine to stop the release of histamine in the body: histamine plays a crucial role in the brain, largely controlling a number of cognitive functions. It helps us to keep alert, to maintain concentration, and to stay awake. If histamine were prevented from working in the body, not only would our allergies disappear, but we would also find it difficult to be attentive, we might fall asleep or generally be more careless and lax. Children and students would find it particularly difficult to keep up in class and be affected especially around exam time. They might end up falling so far behind that they would eventually give up. Adults might experience dangerous repercussions, such as falling asleep at the wheel of the car, failing to operate machinery safely, or making bad decisions that could affect both themselves and others. It is not feasible, therefore, to stop the body's natural production of histamine.

Older versus newer antihistamines

There is plenty of evidence that the older antihistamines are accompanied by some of the above-mentioned effects. For instance, they have been seen to contribute to poor learning in schools, and to road accidents, as they affect the brain in a similar way to alcohol. In a small number of people, they have been known to cause difficulty in urinating, increased pressure in the eyes (glaucoma), cloudiness of the eye lens (cataract), or damage to the cornea, the transparent layer that forms the front of the eye. These eye conditions can all lead to gradual loss of sight. Other possible side effects of these antihistamines include headaches, dry mouth and throat, nausea and digestive problems.

It's fortunate that the newer antihistamines are vastly improved and have been prepared in such a way that they are prevented from reaching the brain from the bloodstream. They are just as efficient in treating hay fever symptoms but have minimal adverse effect on cognitive function.

In general, the older antihistamines such as chlorpheniramine (brand name Piriton) are now only prescribed by doctors in special circumstances. Even very young children, between ages two and five, should not be given the older ones, unless prescribed to induce sleepiness for some reason. One possible reason for inducing sleepiness in a child may be to minimize itching in severe eczema.

If you have been taking one of the older antihistamines for several years, you would be well advised to ask your doctor for one of the newer variety. Unfortunately, the older antihistamines are still on sale over the counter and, due to their lower cost, may appear more attractive. Expert medical opinion would state, however, that drowsiness is an unacceptable side effect and these older drugs should not be used. It is hoped that they are withdrawn from over-the-counter purchase in the near future.

The new antihistamines are considered very safe. Potentially, they can cause the same side effects as the older antihistamines, but they are far less likely to do so. However, when taken in tablet form they can interact with other medications you may be taking, so it is important to mention these when seeing your doctor. Antihistamines also have the potential to interact with alcohol, so it is best to ensure that you drink nothing or very little while taking them. Read the instruction leaflet very carefully.

Usage of antihistamines

Antihistamines are the mainstay of hay fever treatment and certain other allergies. They generally come in tablet form or as a nasal spray and effectively ease symptoms related to the nose and eyes. They can also stop the terrible itching sensations in the throat, soft palate and ears.

However, they are not so useful at relieving nasal blockage, and other medications may have to be used in conjunction with antihistamines.

All in all, the only other hay fever medications that are equally effective are steroid based – in the form of tablet or injection – and immunotherapy (as discussed later in this chapter). Steroidal medications and immunotherapy treatment both carry side effects not shared by antihistamines.

Availability of the newer antihistamines

Antihistamines currently available over the counter in the UK include the following:

- loratadine (brand names Clarityn, Clarityne and Claritin)
- acrivastine (brand names Benadryl, Semprex and Allergy Relief Capsules)
- cetirizine (brand names Zyrtec and Zirtec).

Antihistamines currently available on prescription in the UK include the following:

- fexofenadine (brand names Telfast 120, or Allegra in the USA)
- desloratadine (brand name Neoclarityn)
- mizolastine (brand name Mizollen).

Due to their adverse side effects, two antihistamines, astemizole and terfenadine, have been withdrawn from use in recent years – death from an irregular heartbeat was even a risk. If you still have old supplies in your medicine cabinet, ask your doctor whether it is safe for you to use them. You are likely to be offered a prescription for a newer antihistamine.

Effectiveness and speed of action

As with all medications, the effectiveness of different antihistamines varies, as does the length of time for which it provides relief and the degree of sleepiness it causes, if any. For instance, acrivastine is reported to take effect more rapidly than other antihistamines. Generally, however, the newer antihistamines start working in less than an hour. Acrivastine is different from the rest of its family of medications too in that it is taken three times a day – the others are taken only once a day.

Pregnancy and breastfeeding

Not all of the newer antihistamines have been around for long enough for their effect on unborn babies and breastfeeding babies to be systematically calculated. However, women who have not realized they were pregnant for several months have taken the new antihistamines with no adverse effect to the child. It can be said, therefore, that they have already been safely used by many thousands of pregnant women.

Of course, a small percentage of women will always give birth to babies with a mental or physical disability, and any medications taken during the early stages of pregnancy will always be queried by doctors and parents alike. The fact that there have been no reports of harm to the newborn for the mother taking the new antihistamines has, then, to be a mark of their safety.

It should also be said that the older antihistamines were subjected to rigorous research and there was no evidence of their being a risk to an unborn child – and the newer drugs are all based on their older forebears. For instance, fexofenadine is classed as fairly new, but its commonly used predecessor, terfenadine, is actually converted into fexofenadine in the body. In similar fashion, loratadine, which has been used for a number of years, produces desloratadine in the body, which strongly suggests that the new antihistamine desloratadine will also be safe. If you are pregnant, it is still well worth discussing with your doctor the possible benefits and risks of taking an antihistamine. Great caution in taking any medication will always be advocated, but your doctor is unlikely to want you to put up with difficult symptoms when there is a good available treatment – even though it has a possible tiny (and as yet unrecognized) risk.

As there have been no reports of side effects in a nursing infant, antihistamine medications are also believed to be safe for a breastfeeding mother to take.

Antihistamine nasal sprays

As explained earlier, an excessive amount of histamine and other inflammatory chemicals that occur naturally in the human body are produced from the mast cells when they come into contact with an allergen. The histamine sets up an inflammatory action to rid the body of the allergen, giving rise to the symptoms of hay fever in the process. Antihistamines work by very cleverly rushing to the areas where histamine becomes more active and effectively blocking the inflammatory action.

When antihistamines are delivered by nasal spray, there is usually good symptom relief and many people find that they don't need to take tablets, which get into the whole body. Currently, the only antihistamine available in a nasal spray is azelastin hydrochloride (brand name Astelin), which is obtainable on prescription. Its possible side effects include a bitter taste, headache, nose bleeds, nasal burning, dry mouth, fatigue, dizziness and nausea. As the spray usually takes seven to ten days to reach its maximum effectiveness, it is best to start using it prior to the start of the hay fever season.

As with the antihistamines taken in tablet form, the antihistamine nasal spray is considered safe during pregnancy and breastfeeding.

Anti-allergy agents

There are two main anti-allergy agents – sodium cromoglicate (also referred to as cromolyn and cromoglycate) and nedocromil sodium, both of which are usually very effective and have a good safety record. Sodium cromoglicate comes in the form of nasal spray or eye drops, whereas nedocromil sodium is available as eye drops only. Both work locally to stop the allergen from stimulating an allergic reaction.

Before using any anti-allergy medication, you should inform your doctor if you are pregnant or planning a pregnancy and ask for advice. Because the benefits to a pregnant woman with severe hay fever are likely to exceed the slight risk to the unborn child, anti-allergy agents are recommended when absolutely necessary. Your doctor will be able to offer you individual advice.

Although it is not known whether either sodium cromoglicate or nedocromil sodium passes into breast milk, experts anticipate no problems for the child. Even so, it is recommended that you seek medical advice before using this medication during breastfeeding.

Sodium cromoglicate

This agent is capable of halting the release of histamine and other inflammatory chemicals from the mast cells. It is therefore also classified as an anti-inflammatory drug. Exactly how it manages to stop the release of histamine is not as yet fully understood, but it somehow stabilizes the mast cells so they don't react by releasing their chemicals. Medications containing sodium cromoglicate are fairly short-acting so generally require up to four applications in a day. For the very best results, they need to be used approximately two weeks in advance of symptoms appearing, but if symptoms are already in evidence anti-allergy agents can prevent them from getting any worse and still provide a lot of relief.

Although anti-allergy agents are often less effective than nasal corticosteroids (discussed later in this chapter), they are generally the medication of choice for young children.

Sodium cromoglicate nasal spray

This anti-allergy nasal spray is very good for relieving symptoms related to the nose, such as sneezing, excessive production of mucus, itching and nasal congestion. The sodium cromoglicate nasal sprays available include Rynacrom, Nasalcrom or Resiston 1. It's important to note that this type of nasal spray should be used for only four weeks after first opening the container. After that it should be thrown away or returned to your chemist. It may be helpful to write the date of opening on the box. If you are aware of an allergy to any of the ingredients in the medication, inform your doctor or pharmacist immediately.

Although there have been no reports of birth defects in a newborn, or side effects in a nursing infant, this type of nasal spray should be used with caution if you are pregnant or breastfeeding. If your symptoms are severe, your doctor may recommend this treatment and carefully monitor your progress.

Sodium cromoglicate eye drops

These anti-allergy eye drops are usually very good for easing sore, watery eyes and other eye symptoms related to hay fever. Eye symptoms are actually referred to as allergic conjunctivitis, or even 'hay fever eyes'. The drops are available under the brand names of Optrex Allergy, Opticrom, Clariteyes, Hay-crom or Crolom, and are most effective when used regularly, even when symptoms are slight or have temporarily disappeared.

Nedocromil sodium eye drops

Nedocromil sodium is a newer type of anti-allergy agent, available on prescription in the form of eye drops under the brand name of Rapitil. Start using the drops approximately two weeks before the onset of symptoms, applying twice daily for maximum relief.

As with sodium cromoglicate medications, there have been no reports of birth defects in a newborn, or side effects in a nursing infant while the mother was using nedocromil sodium eye drops. However, caution should still be employed as with any medication.

Decongestants

Decongestants can be taken in tablet form, as nasal sprays and as eye drops. They can be a very good treatment for the stuffiness that often occurs in hay fever, but should be used with great caution. When used for longer than three days a 'rebound' condition known as rhinitis medicamentosa can occur, in which increased congestion can make it difficult to breathe through the nose. You then have no choice but to stop using the medication immediately and wait until the situation improves by itself, putting up with severe stuffiness until you return to the state you were in before you started using it.

If you are pregnant or planning to become pregnant, it's important to seek your doctor's advice before taking decongestants of any kind. The same applies for a woman who is breastfeeding.

Oral decongestants

Although decongestants in tablet form can certainly help to unblock the nose and sinuses, they should also be taken for no more than three days, for the same above-mentioned reasons. There is also evidence of a very slight risk of potentially serious side effects. For instance, it has been found that one oral decongestant, called phenylpropanolamine, can cause strokes as a result of bleeding in the brain, especially in a person with high blood pressure. It can also give rise to problems in people with diabetes, thyroid problems or heart disease.

When a decongestant is combined with an antihistamine in tablet form, tests have shown that they work very well on a short-term basis. Some oral decongestants combined with an antihistamine can be purchased over the counter, but you are strongly advised to ask your doctor to recommend the most suitable one for you. The potential risks of taking phenylpropanolamine have diminished the enthusiasm for this drug, and another fact to be considered is that oral decongestants can interact with other medications such as those for depression or Parkinson's disease.

Decongestant nasal sprays

Decongestant sprays with the ingredient oxymetazoline hydrochloride (brand names Afrin, Vicks and Sinex), which are effective for less severe symptoms, can be bought directly from chemists and some supermarkets. For short-term use, they are far safer than oral decongestants, and work by constricting blood vessels in the lining of the nose, rapidly opening up the nasal passages, reducing congestion and making it easier to breathe. As the medicine in the spray is localized to the nose, there is less risk of side effects occurring. When a course of hay fever treatment begins, just before the start of the hay fever season, doctors often recommend the short-term use of a decongestant spray in combination with an antihistamine or steroidal spray. This is because the rapid action of the decongestant enables the other sprays to be more effective.

Note that decongestant sprays should be used for no longer than three days, as longer usage can make a blocked nose more blocked, as mentioned above. Steroidal and antihistamine sprays don't have this side effect.

Decongestant eye drops

To give fast relief for itchy, watery eyes, decongestant eye drops may be used. After application, you may experience temporary stinging or burning in the eyes, but this should soon disappear. If you encounter any other side effects, such as eye irritation, headache, cough, dry mouth and nausea, it is best to stop using the drops and seek your doctor's advice.

As with other types of decongestant, the eye drops should not be used for more than three consecutive days, to prevent the onset of rebound congestion.

Corticosteroidal medications

Medications containing corticosteroids – often referred to simply as 'steroids' – can effectively regulate immune system function, suppressing the inflammatory response and giving fast relief. As a result, they work very well, but should only be used when all else fails and something stronger is required to deal with severe symptoms. Corticosteroids are available only on prescription from your doctor, who will carefully explain the warnings and special precautions attached to them.

Although there have been no adequate trials into the effects of corticosteroids in pregnancy, recent analysis of data suggests a small but significant link between corticosteroids taken in the first trimester (three months) of pregnancy and cleft palate in the newborn. It is advisable, therefore, to avoid corticosteroids during pregnancy. There is no available data into the effects of corticosteroids when breastfeeding, so it is best to ask your doctor's advice.

Corticosteroidal tablets

Corticosteroids in tablet form are powerful drugs for the treatment of severe hay fever. They may not remove every last symptom, but they can make life a lot more bearable and are particularly useful for allowing you to function more normally in important life events, such as exams, weddings, interviews and so on.

The steroid used in hay fever medications is not of the type used by athletes to enhance their performance, with notorious side effects – that is, anabolic steroids. However, if not administered within the proper guidelines they do carry the slight risk of the following adverse effects:

- increased appetite and weight gain
- water and salt retention leading to swelling
- fat deposits in the face, chest, stomach and upper back
- high blood pressure
- increased susceptibility to infection
- diabetes
- cataracts
- acne
- depression
- muscle weakness.

To minimize the possible occurrence of side effects, it will probably be recommended that you take only a low dose of this oral drug for a very short period. Your doctor will doubtlessly monitor your progress very carefully and ask you to stop taking the drug once the crisis or important event is over.

While taking corticosteroids, it is safe to use other hay fever treatments.

Corticosteroidal injections

If you have severe symptoms that fail to respond to other treatments, it is possible to have a corticosteroidal injection. Unlike corticosteroidal tablets which are effective for only the short period of time you take them, the injection administers what doctors call 'depot steroids' that remain active for a longer time, whether you still require them to be in your body or not. The injection comes with all the risk factors of tablet-form corticosteroids; in addition it can cause 'fat atrophy', in which a dent in your buttock appears where the injection was delivered. In rare cases an abscess can occur at the injection site.

A corticosteroidal injection administered when hay fever symptoms first appear can give symptom remission that lasts for the duration of the entire pollen season. However, due to the many possible side effects associated with corticosteroids (as listed above) doctors will offer the injection only as a last resort.

Corticosteroidal nasal sprays

Corticosteroidal sprays – sometimes referred to as 'sticky sprays' – have anti-inflammatory properties and effectively reduce swelling and congestion in the sinuses and nasal cavities, without causing drowsiness. Moreover, when used in the nose, this steroidal drug is actually very safe and works better than any other spray.

Corticosteroidal nasal sprays are even believed to be safe for long-term use. This is due to the following:

- The dosage of steroidal medicine in a nasal spray is very low.
- The medicine in the spray breaks down very quickly in the body, not allowing sufficient time for side effects to arise.
- In the past doctors were concerned that prolonged use of a steroidal nasal spray would make the nose lining very thin. However, time has shown that the lining is actually healthier after long-term steroidal use than it would have been after prolonged inflammation.

As with most nasal sprays that are aimed at treating hay fever, using this medication can cause an inflamed nose to sting for a while. If this happens, try to persevere with the spray for a few days, and the membranes should gradually become less swollen. In a small percentage of people, unfortunately, the stinging may continue. Seek your doctor's advice if this happens to you.

Some people find sufficient relief from using a corticosteroidal nasal spray and don't need to take tablets, which get into the whole body. If you can't help worrying about the effects of using steroids, even in a spray, you may find that an antihistamine spray is equally effective. As with most other hay fever treatments, more benefit is gained from using it early – for about two weeks prior to the start of the hay fever season. This stops the inflammation from building up. For maximum benefit, the spray must then be used on a daily basis for the duration of the hay fever season.

There are two available over-the-counter preparations – beclomethasone (brand name Beconase) and fluticasone (brand name Flonase). Other corticosteroidal nasal sprays are available on prescription only.

Although there have been no adequately controlled trials into the effects of corticosteroidal nasal sprays in pregnancy, there have also been no reports of resultant birth defects. However, caution is always advisable when thinking of taking medications during pregnancy and breastfeeding. Ask your doctor's advice if you are unsure of what to do.

Corticosteroidal eye drops

Unfortunately, corticosteroids have many possible disadvantages when used in the eye, such as impairing the ability of the eye to fight infections and repair itself after injury. Glaucoma (increase in pressure in the eye), cataracts and eventual loss of vision can also occur. For these reasons, such drops should be used in only very severe cases, in people whose eyes have become very itchy, inflamed, watery and bloodshot, and when no other eye treatment has proved effective. They can, however, make a great difference. Like the steroidal nasal spray, the best results come from using eye drops shortly before the hay fever season gets under way.

These eye drops should only be used in pregnancy and breastfeeding if the potential benefit outweighs the possible risk. Ask your doctor about this.

Saline nasal sprays

Nasal sprays containing only saline – a solution of salt in water – can be a useful temporary treatment for people with hay fever. A regular squirt of the solution into dry and irritated nostrils may ease the discomfort by moisturizing the area. Saline sprays are available over-the-counter from most chemists.

Tips for using oral medications

The following can help you to get the most from medications in tablet or capsule form:

- Read the packet instruction leaflet very carefully before starting the medication.
- Give the medication you are offered a chance to work. It may take several days for real benefits to be seen. Remember, though, that decongestants must not be used for more than three days.
- If you experience unacceptable side effects, stop the treatment and go to your doctor.
- If you are aware of an allergy to any of the ingredients in the medication, inform your doctor or pharmacist immediately.
- From time to time, ask your doctor whether improved medications with fewer side effects have become available.
- Ask that your allergy status be assessed periodically so that any new allergies can be treated.

Tips for using nasal sprays

The nose can become very inflamed and sore in hay fever, and continual exposure to the same levels of pollen can in fact appear to make nasal symptoms progressively worse. Nasal sprays can alleviate nasal congestion and therefore prevent this decline. Most nasal sprays deliver a fine mist, containing appropriate medications, into the nostril by means of a miniature hand-pump mechanism. It is common for a doctor or allergy specialist to prescribe a combination of nasal sprays, or nasal sprays combined with other medications.

As mentioned earlier, some nasal sprays may cause a temporary stinging sensation on application, particularly if the area is very inflamed. After a few days, however, the inflammation should be reduced and the sensation should ease. Some people are unable to stand the stinging and prefer to take their hay fever medication in tablet or capsule form only. Not all nasal sprays sting, though, and it is worth experimenting with different brands to find the most suitable for you. Ask your doctor, allergy specialist or pharmacist about this.

A nasal spray should be discarded four weeks after first opening the container, or returned to your pharmacy. It may be helpful to write the date of opening on the box. If you are aware of an allergy to any of the ingredients in the medication, inform your doctor or pharmacist immediately. If you experience side effects other than stinging after using a nasal spray, inform your doctor. In addition, it is important that you read the information sheet provided with the medication.

For optimum relief

As the nose is a complicated, walnut-like arrangement of delicate membranes, it's not easy to cover every bit of it with a spray – especially when you have only two small holes through which to apply it. Indeed, some people have given up trying using nasal sprays because they didn't apply them correctly and found that they weren't any real help. You can obtain maximum benefit by taking note of the following:

1 If need be, blow your nose before using the spray.
2 Bow your head forward and hold the spray at the first nostril so that it is pointing vertically upwards.
3 While sniffing up, squirt one or two puffs into one nostril. Then repeat with the other nostril.
4 Quickly get into a position which places your head upside-down.

This enables the liquid to cover a much wider area. You may wish to kneel with your head between your knees or tilt it backwards over the edge of your bed. Ask a family member to help you, if need be.

5 To spread the liquid around further, sniff in and out rapidly for up to a minute.

6 Get up.

You will know that you are carrying out the procedure correctly if the liquid stops trickling down your throat, like it did previously. If there is indeed no trickle, it has remained in the nose, which is where it is meant to be.

Tips for using eye drops

It is advisable to follow these tips before using eye drops:

- Eye drops should be applied directly to your eye using the dropper provided. They should not be taken by mouth.
- To avoid contamination, be careful to avoid touching the tip of the dropper to any surface, including your eye.
- After application, the drops may temporarily blur your vision. It is therefore important not to drive or operate machinery until the blurring has cleared completely.
- If you normally use contact lenses, wear glasses instead for the duration of your treatment. Most eye drops contain a preservative that can irritate the eye.
- Eye drops should be thrown away or returned to your pharmacy four weeks after first opening the container. It may be helpful to write the date of opening on the box.
- If you are aware of an allergy to any of the ingredients in the medication, inform your doctor or chemist immediately.
- If your eyes are inflamed, applying eye drops can cause them to sting a little for a while. You shouldn't worry unnecessarily about this. The reason for the stinging is not the medicine itself, but the germ-killing antiseptic added to make them as safe as possible – some eye drops are used for other eye problems besides hay fever. After a few days, when the drops start taking effect, they should not sting nearly so much. If you are unable to cope with the stinging you may prefer to take your hay fever medication in tablet form instead, which can be equally effective, but with an increased potential for side effects (see pages 47–55).

- If you experience further side effects from using eye drops, inform your doctor. It is important that you read the information sheet provided with the medication.
- If you are using more than one type of eye drop, the second type may wash away the first if administered immediately afterwards. It is therefore essential to leave an interval of at least five minutes between applications. Any eye gels or ointments you are using should be applied last of all.

Immunotherapy

A last resort treatment for people with severe and persistent hay fever, whose symptoms are proving impossible to control and who find it difficult to lead normal lives, may be a treatment regime called immunotherapy, also sometimes known as desensitization. Immunotherapy focuses on training the body to dampen down its production of antibodies when faced with a substance it sees as an invader (the allergen). Other allergy treatments are aimed at reducing the symptoms of allergic disease, but immunotherapy is actually capable of reducing the body's sensitivity to allergens. As a result, the course of the disease is often automatically modified, providing long-term symptom relief.

You should seek advice from an allergy specialist prior to embarking on immunotherapy. The specialist will attempt to ensure that you are a suitable candidate who will definitely benefit from this expensive and time-consuming treatment and who is not at risk of possible adverse allergic reaction. If you are referred to an allergy specialist to discuss the possibility of immunotherapy, it is a great opportunity for you to also gather advice about other treatments. You may even then decide that you would prefer to give other treatments another try rather than undergo the prolonged regime of immunotherapy.

If you and the allergy specialist decide that immunotherapy is your best option, you will begin an individually tailored three- to five-year programme of weekly or fortnightly injections – referred to as vaccinations or 'allergy shots' – starting just before the hay fever season commences. The injections are virtually pain-free and carried out in a hospital environment, to enable you to receive swift and proper attention should you experience a life-threatening allergic reaction. You will be introduced to tiny dilute amounts of the problematic substance – called an allergy extract – to which you are known to be allergic; that is, the particular pollens and moulds. Your response is closely monitored for about an hour after the injection. If your response is manageable, progressively larger doses of the allergen are delivered over your next treatments, and this allows your body to adjust to the allergen and see it as less of a threat – this process is called desensitization. The eventual aim is for the severity of symptoms to be reduced, hopefully drastically and for many years to come. If you miss appointments, however, the dose of the next injection will require modification and consequently the total length of the programme will be extended.

When the injections are administered by an expert, side effects are rare. However, temporary swelling or itchiness at the site – known as allergen resistance – is occasionally experienced. If this happens, you are likely to be offered an antihistamine shortly before the next injection is due.

In a range of studies, immunotherapy has exhibited its ability to give long-term benefits for existing allergies. It has also been shown to be capable of modifying the development of any new allergies and even of reducing the risk of developing asthma. However, this treatment is not an absolute cure, it does not offer benefit for everyone and for some people it is effective to only a very small degree. Still, most people who have undergone immunotherapy find that their symptoms are more bearable and also more responsive to other treatments. Some even find that it allows them eventually to stop taking their allergy medication.

International guidelines on injection immunotherapy, revised in 2007, confirmed the clinical efficacy of this technique for treating hay fever and asthma. Provided that the guideline recommendations are adhered to, its safety was also established. Immunotherapy is now seen as a suitable treatment for children with severe hay fever as it also reduces the risk of asthma onset. Indeed, studies have shown that the earlier in life the treatment begins after an allergy reveals itself, the more chance there is of success.

In the UK, immunotherapy is often a last-resort treatment because of its expense to the National Health Service. However, in the long term both patients and the NHS make savings on the cost of medications. It is to be hoped, therefore, that immunotherapy is soon made more widely available.

Interestingly, there is now a sublingual (placed under the tongue) tablet containing a grass pollen extract that can be taken at home without the need for injections, specialist doctors and medical centres. The tablet appears to be as effective as immunotherapy and has few side effects. It is now being offered to people with asthma who are not suitable candidates for injection immunotherapy.

6

Self-treatment for hay fever

Many people with hay fever are able successfully to treat themselves at home without medication, usually by using a combination of techniques. The obvious way to eliminate symptoms is to avoid the substance that is causing the problem, which is, unfortunately, easier said than done. Moreover, the exact allergens responsible are not always apparent. Even allergy specialists are sometimes unable to determine the exact culprits, in which case self-treatment can be an invaluable aid.

How to control hay fever symptoms

To reduce or even prevent inflammation of the tissues affected in hay fever, there are plenty of things you can do. Here are some basic recommendations:

- Stay indoors when the outdoor pollen count is at its highest, in the morning and evening – particularly between 5 p.m. and 7 p.m. if you live in or near the countryside and a couple of hours later if you live in an urban area. The peak pollen time is not the hottest part of the day but later on, when airborne pollen starts to fall towards the ground.
- If you live or work on a high floor in a tall block of flats or offices, ensure that the windows are closed in the middle of the day. Pollen rises in the atmosphere and is more likely to enter through high windows earlier in the day than it would in a lower building.
- When indoors, keep all doors and windows closed during the evening and night at high pollen times. If the weather is hot, use an air-conditioning system if possible, or if you don't have this, draw the curtains before the sun gets too hot, to block out the heat and keep the temperature down.
- If you must spend time outdoors, consider wearing a mask that is designed to filter out pollen. A retailer of pollen masks is listed in Useful addresses at the back of this book.
- Unless you are wearing a pollen mask, don't cycle or walk through areas you know set off your symptoms, such as fields, parks, woods

and large grassy areas. Instead, use a contained means of transport, such as a car, a bus or even a train.

- If you have to be anywhere near long grass and trees, consider wearing a mask and either prescription spectacles if you have them, green-tinted glasses, wraparound sunglasses or goggles. It is better to look a little silly than suffer the misery of hay fever symptoms.
- To soothe a sore throat, gargle with warm salty water. Dissolve 1–2 tablespoons of table salt into 200 ml (8 fl oz) of warm water.
- When in the car, keep the windows closed. Use air-conditioning if you have it, and consider buying a pollen filter for the air vents.
- Don't have fresh flowers in the house, or close to you at work. Make it clear to family and friends that while flowers as a gift are lovely, they make your hay fever worse.
- Dust your furniture with a damp cloth rather than a dry duster, which will help to prevent dust and pollen particles from flying into the air.
- Damp dust and vacuum your home as often as possible. Consider buying a vacuum cleaner with a HEPA filter.
- Avoid eating any foods to which you know you are sensitive (see 'Oral allergy syndrome' on page 27) – they may aggravate your hay fever symptoms.
- If possible, ask someone else to mow the lawn, rake the leaves and prune the bushes.
- To prevent any pollen that has attached itself to you from entering your nose, frequently wash your hands and face. When you come in the house from outside, change your clothes.
- If there is about to be a thunderstorm, stay inside with the windows closed. Changes in atmospheric pressure can break down pollens into very fine particles which are more easily inhaled.
- When thinking of holidays, consider going to the coast as sea breezes blow pollen inland.
- Go sightseeing outside of the peak pollen season.
- Take regular note of the pollen count, which is usually broadcast on TV and radio along with the weather.

If your hay fever is severe, there are several more 'exacting' rules you could follow to achieve optimum relief from your symptoms.

- You may find it worth investing in an air-conditioning system or HEPA filter at home. This will remove most of the pollen and other allergens from the air around you.

- Wipe down your dog or cat with a damp towel after they have been outdoors. They may have picked up pollen from the air.
- Place a thin layer of petroleum jelly (such as Vaseline) around your eyes and just inside the nostrils to prevent pollen from entering these areas.
- Before you go to bed, take a shower to remove any pollen that is stuck to your body or hair.
- Avoid drying your clothes, towels and bed linen outdoors.
- Avoid exposing yourself to other environmental irritants such as chemical fumes, fly spray, strong perfumes, paint, fresh tar and tobacco smoke.
- When planning your garden, choose plants that give off the least amount of pollen. Alternatively, have your garden tiled or gravelled over (see Chapter 9 for more information on low-allergen gardening).
- Spray a fine mist of water over the garden with the hose to dampen down pollen in the air.
- If you can, avoid living near to a busy road where there are high levels of vehicle exhaust fumes or to an industrial estate where chemical pollutants are sure to be circulating in the air. Moving to a less polluted area would significantly reduce your allergens.
- If your symptoms are bad at night, use an ionizer in the bedroom, which may help you get a better night's sleep.
- Consider colon cleansing to detoxify your intestines. The effect can be a substantial reduction in allergy symptoms.

During a hay fever flare-up, avoid hot drinks as these can increase blood flow to the nasal membranes, causing further inflammation. If you are suffering from hives (urticaria), you can purchase antihistamine creams or steroid preparations from high street chemists. Regular application, in accordance with the instruction leaflet, should relieve the itchiness.

How to make yourself feel better

The recommendations given in this section can help make life with hay fever far more bearable.

Fresh air and sunlight

If your hay fever is bad, you will obviously try to avoid being outdoors during high pollen times (such as in the morning and evening). It is important, however, that you don't lock yourself away indoors all the time. Fresh air and sunlight are vital to good health for the following reasons:

- Fresh air helps to dispel toxic gases from our bodies, via the lungs.
- Clean, fresh oxygen helps to sustain the metabolic reactions within every cell in our bodies.
- Sunlight provides our bodies with important vitamins, such as vitamin D which helps to keep our bones strong – this is important if you are reducing your consumption of cow's milk products (see Chapter 7 for nutritional advice).

Exercise

If at all possible, carrying out a daily exercise routine, or being involved in recreational activities such as football, swimming or tennis will help.

- Exercise reduces your levels of stress – and stress is one of the exacerbating factors in hay fever.
- It stimulates the lymph glands, which operate as a sewage system to rid the body of harmful toxins. The flow of lymph (a clear fluid containing white blood cells) from the lymph glands is entirely dependent upon muscular movement.
- Regular exercise can also increase the body's tolerance of chemicals in the environment.
- Exercise floods your body with endorphins – the natural feel-good chemicals that give you a 'lift'.

Get plenty of sleep

A good night's sleep will help to reduce the feelings of fatigue and lassitude common during a hay fever attack. If you find that your symptoms are keeping you awake and that you are sleeping far less than the usual seven or eight hours, speak to your doctor. You may require stronger medication. There are also herbal remedies, such as Herbal Nytol, that may help you to get a better night's sleep. If you are seeing a complementary health therapist, such as a homeopath, hypnotherapist or reflexologist, do mention if you are not sleeping very well and they will incorporate a treatment for this into their therapy programme.

Take hot baths and saunas

If possible, have a sauna at least once a week – the steam can help to alleviate your symptoms. There are saunas now at most swimming baths and recreation centres. It's often particularly helpful to use a portable facial sauna, which can be purchased from certain specialist manufacturers.

Taking a hot bath at least once a day, rather than showering, can help you to feel better.

Use honey to immunize yourself against pollen

To help desensitize your body to pollen, try taking a daily table-spoon of raw honey – produced locally, if possible, so that it is likely to contain the pollens to which you are allergic. Add a little fresh bee pollen – available from most health food shops – starting with one or two granules and gradually increasing to half a tablespoon. It is important to monitor your reaction very carefully and be ready to reduce temporarily the amount if your symptoms worsen.

Nasal irrigation

You may have heard that nasal irrigation – rinsing out the nostrils with salty water – can reduce inflammation of the mucous mem-branes. This procedure is not always of benefit, however, as it can alter the nasal environment and encourage the growth of water-loving bac-teria such as pseudomonas. Moreover, if used to treat acute sinusitis, nasal irrigation can actually spread the infection to the throat, eyes or other sinuses. As you may have acute sinusitis but not be aware of it, it is important to carry out the procedure only when advised to do so by your doctor.

If your doctor recommends you to try it, the procedure involves inhaling the solution (detailed below). Inhaling can be achieved either by holding the solution in a cupped hand and sniffing it up through your nose, or by using a small bulb syringe – sold in most chemists – to inject the solution up each nostril in turn, as deeply as possible. It is quite normal for some of it to run down the back of your throat. Use the solution as instructed, probably two to three times a day.

Prepare 1 pint (560 ml) of solution at a time and store it in a clean air-tight container. If the solution begins to look cloudy or there is matter floating in it, throw it away and make a fresh batch. The solu-tion should contain:

- 1 teaspoon of salt
- 1 teaspoon of baking soda (not baking powder)
- 1 pint (560 ml) of pre-boiled warm water.

Herbal remedies

A number of herbal remedies are recognized as being useful in treating hay fever symptoms. If you are at all unsure of how to prepare and use them, don't hesitate to consult an experienced herbalist, who will ensure that you are obtaining the most suitable remedies and offer step-by-step guidance. A herbalist will also be able to prescribe more potent remedies that are not on general sale.

The herbs mentioned here are available from most health food shops, usually as dried herbs or in tincture form. Follow the dosage instructions unless otherwise advised.

Elderflower

Elderflower is a particularly useful preventative remedy. The astringent action of the organic substances called tannins it contains helps to dry up a runny nose and watery eyes, reducing inflammation in the process. Starting in February or March and continuing right through the hay fever season, drink one cup of elderflower infusion daily. In season, you can pick elderflowers from hedgerows – but be careful not to take them from areas where agricultural chemicals may have been used. The fresh flowers of the plant work best, but when they are not in flower you can buy them in dried form from herbalists and some health food shops. Alternatively, use elderflower tincture or a good-quality elderflower cordial.

Adding ribwort plantain (see below) to your infusion can strengthen the mucous membranes of the nasal passages and help to make them less sensitive to allergens. Dried plantain is available from herbalists and some health food shops. It also comes in tincture form.

If you intend collecting elderflower yourself, make sure you are certain what plants you are picking. Some wildflowers and other plants are poisonous.

For elderflower cordial you will need:

- 25 heads of elderflower, rinsed
- 2 kg of soft brown sugar
- 2 litres of water
- 2 lemons, sliced.

Place the sugar, water and lemons in a saucepan and heat up, stirring all the time until the sugar dissolves. Allow to cool, then pour over the elderflowers. Allow to stand in a covered container for two days, then strain and pour into bottles. Secure the bottles with corks, then store in a cool, dark place. To drink, dilute one part of the cordial to three parts of water. If you prefer elderflower 'champagne', dilute with sparkling mineral water.

Nettle

Nettle is a natural antihistamine. Taking it in tea infusions or as a juice can reduce the inflammation produced by the body during an allergic reaction. It is therefore able to ease nasal congestion, watery eyes, chest congestion and many of the other symptoms related to hay fever.

Ingesting nettle on a regular basis – as much as four times a day – can gradually desensitize you to the effects of pollen. It may be possible to obtain fresh or dried nettle leaves from a herbalist; if you chew them during an allergic attack there can be immediate beneficial effects.

Echinacea

One of the most researched of all herbs, echinacea has broad antibiotic properties, a bit like penicillin. It also has the effect of strengthening the immune system, deterring it from mistakenly identifying innocuous substances as enemy forces. This effectively reduces the body's sensitivity to allergens. Echinacea works best used in combination with goldenseal, red clover and sage, which cleanse the blood and lymph (a clear fluid containing white blood cells which bathes the tissues) of the toxic metabolites that arise during an allergic response.

Alcohol-free tinctures are now available from most health food shops. Dry echinacea root – also available from health food shops – can be infused to make tea.

Goldenseal

Like elderflower, goldenseal has astringent properties which can help to reduce eye watering and the production of nasal mucus. It is particularly beneficial when taken with echinacea for soothing the mucous membranes, and can effectively relieve symptoms where sinusitis or sinus infection is present.

Red clover

Red clover is a blood and lymph cleanser, helping to remove the toxic waste which arises during an allergic reaction. It therefore has a therapeutic effect on hay fever symptoms.

This herb should not be used during pregnancy and breastfeeding.

Sage

To soothe an itchy throat and palate, gargle daily with a herbal infusion of sage. This herb also acts as a blood and lymph cleanser, much like red clover. When combined with echinacea, hay fever symptoms can be greatly reduced.

Ma huang (Chinese ephedra)

This herb is often used in the treatment of asthma and hay fever. It contains ephedrine – an alkaloid obtained from the ephedra (an evergreen shrub) which actively constricts the blood vessels and widens the bronchial passages. It is therefore useful for controlling the acute symptoms of hay fever such as a streaming nose and sinus congestion.

It is important to note that this herb should not be used for more than a week at a time. Longer usage can cause overstimulation of the central nervous system.

Rhodiola rosea

This powerful Russian nutrient belongs to the family of adaptogenic herbs, which encourages the body to adapt to stress. Research has shown that rhodiola rosea has a protective effect on the immune system: it helps to raise energy levels, it increases resistance to disease and it aids detoxification.

Siberian ginseng

The many benefits of Siberian ginseng – the best known of the adaptogenic herbs – include increased physical endurance under stress, protection against infection, improved immune system function and improved hormone activity. It can therefore be of benefit in the treatment of hay fever.

Camomile

If your eyes are red, sore and streaming, frequent bathing with a cooled infusion of camomile can be enormously soothing. When the infusion is drunk on a regular basis, it reduces nasal congestion and can lower the nervous system excitability often linked with allergic conditions.

Ribwort plantain

The ribwort variety of plantain can help to reduce inflammation and tone the mucous membranes. Take three times daily as a tea infusion.

Curcumin

This herb is an extract of turmeric and can be used as an anti-inflammatory agent in hay fever. In fact, in a series of trials, it was shown to be as beneficial as prescription cortisone.

Calendula, rosemary oil and thyme oil

To soothe the mucous membranes, rinse the nostrils with solutions of any of these herbal oils. They can also be used as salves in the facial area, such as around the nose and eyes.

Horsetail

Tea infusions of horsetail can also be used to rinse out the nostrils for a soothing effect.

Garlic

Garlic is another immune system strengthener (and see Chapter 7 for inclusion in your diet). Use it in your diet as much as possible, and take it in supplement form, preferably enteric-coated tablets of dried or powdered garlic for optimum benefit.

If you are diabetic or suffer from hypoglycaemia, consult your doctor before taking garlic supplements as they can raise or lower blood sugar levels.

Acidophilus

The probiotic acidophilus is a 'friendly' bacterium found naturally in good-quality yogurts and some other natural foods. After you have taken a course of antibiotics, acidophilus helps to restore the balance of good microflora in the gut, deterring the growth and proliferation of unhealthy bacteria and further infections. Acidophilus is available in probiotic drinks such as Actimel and Yakult, and in supplement form from health food shops.

Ground ivy

This herb is useful in treating hay fever as it can reduce the production of excess catarrh. Use 20–30 drops of the tincture per dose, and take this three times a day.

Feverfew

This herb is believed to have anti-allergenic properties. Indeed, it has been shown in trials to inhibit the release of histamine from the mast cells. Drink daily as a tea infusion or take in capsule form.

Eyebright

This herb (also called euphrasia) is an immune system strengthener and is excellent for reducing nasal secretions and watering eyes. It can also soothe the mucous membranes.

Aloe vera juice

Like yogurt, the juice from the aloe vera plant has mild antihistamine properties. Dilute the juice in water, following the label instructions which will tell you how much to drink and how often. Aloe vera juice is available from some health food shops and specialist outlets (see Useful addresses at the back of this book for suppliers). As a topical gel, aloe vera is also good for treating allergic skin rashes such as eczema.

Liquorice root

A popular remedy for allergy relief, liquorice (or licorice) root has a strengthening effect on the adrenal glands, which are believed to be exhausted in hay fever. It also reduces inflammation. Take liquorice root extract during the hay fever season for symptom relief.

Note that you should avoid this herb if you suffer from high blood pressure or water retention.

Relaxation

Stress is weakening to both the immune system and the adrenal glands. You may even have noticed that your allergy symptoms worsen when you are feeling stressed. Having to deal with hay fever symptoms for several weeks – or even months – at a time doesn't help. Indeed, it can lead to chronic stress – the state of being constantly 'on alert'. The physiological changes associated with this state, which include raised heart-rate, shallow breathing and muscular tension, can even persist after the attack is over, leading to nerviness, hypertension, irritability and depression.

Deep breathing

In normal breathing, we take oxygen from the atmosphere down into our lungs. The diaphragm contracts and air is pulled into the chest cavity. When we breathe out, we expel carbon dioxide and other waste gases back into the atmosphere. But when we are stressed or upset, we tend to use the rib muscles to expand the chest. We breathe more quickly, sucking in shallowly. This is excellent in a crisis, as it allows us to obtain the optimum amount of oxygen in the shortest possible time, providing our bodies with the extra power needed to handle the emergency. However, it can be easy to get stuck in chest-breathing mode. Long-term shallow breathing is not only detrimental to physical and emotional health, it can also lead to hyperventilation, panic attacks, chest pains, dizziness and gastrointestinal problems.

To test your breathing, ask yourself:

- How fast are you breathing as you are reading this?
- Are you pausing between breaths?
- Are you breathing with your chest or with your diaphragm?

A breathing exercise

The following deep-breathing exercise should, ideally, be performed daily.

1 Ensure that you are not wearing tight clothing, and if necessary change into something loose-fitting.
2 Make yourself comfortable in a warm room where you know you will be alone for at least half an hour.
3 Close your eyes and try to relax.
4 Gradually slow down your breathing, inhaling and exhaling as evenly as possible.
5 Place one hand on your chest and the other on your abdomen, just below your ribcage. As you inhale, allow your abdomen to swell upwards. Your chest should barely move.
6 As you exhale, let your abdomen flatten.
7 Give yourself a few minutes to get into a smooth, easy rhythm. As worries and distractions arise, don't hang on to them. Wait calmly for them to float out of your mind, then focus once more on your breathing.

When you feel ready to end the exercise, open your eyes. Allow yourself time to become alert before getting up. With practice, you will begin breathing with your diaphragm quite naturally – and in times of stress, you should be able to correct your breathing without too much effort.

Stress-busting suggestions

In hay fever, stress management should be a high priority. Fortunately, there are many ways to reduce stress, some of which are listed below. If you can carry out two or three (at least) of these suggestions every day, you should find yourself more able to cope with your symptoms, as well as with the difficulties that arise in everyday life.

- Smile as often as you can.
- Drive in the slow lane.
- Perform your daily activities at a slower pace – walking, eating, reading, housework, washing the car, doing the crossword puzzle and so on.
- Stop yourself from grimacing.
- Buy a small gift for someone you care about.
- Tell someone you care about how much they mean to you.
- Refer to yourself less frequently in conversation.
- Practise controlling your anger.
- Pay someone a compliment.
- Allow yourself to cry if you feel like doing so.
- Practise assertiveness.
- Listen to music.
- Take a long bath.
- Alter your routine slightly.

A relaxation exercise

Relaxation is one of the forgotten skills in today's hectic world, but it can help to counter the effects of stress arising from hay fever symptoms. It's advisable, therefore, that you learn at least one relaxation technique. The following exercise is perhaps the easiest:

1 Ensure that you are not wearing tight clothing.
2 Make yourself comfortable in a place where you will not be disturbed. Listening to restful music may help you relax.
3 Begin to slow down your breathing, inhaling through your nose to a count of two.
4 Ensuring that the abdomen pushes outwards (as explained above), exhale to a count of four, five or six.

After a couple of minutes, concentrate on each part of your body in turn, starting with your right arm. Consciously relax each set of muscles, allowing the tension to flow right out. Let your arm feel heavier and heavier as every last remnant of tension seeps away.

Follow this procedure with the muscles of your left arm, then the muscles of your face, your neck, your stomach, your hips, and finally your legs.

Visualization

At this point visualization can be introduced into the exercise. As you continue to breathe slowly and evenly, imagine yourself on a deserted tropical beach, listening to the sounds of the ocean, thousands of miles from your worries and cares. Let the warm sun, the gentle breeze, the peacefulness of it all wash over you.

The tranquillity you feel at this stage can be enhanced by repeating the relaxation exercise frequently – once or twice a day is best. With time, you should be able to switch into a calm state of mind whenever you feel stressed.

Meditation

Arguably the oldest natural therapy, meditation is the simplest and most effective form of self-help. Dr Herbert Benson of Harvard Medical School has shown that meditation tends to normalize blood pressure, the pulse rate and level of stress hormones in the blood. He has proved, too, that it produces changes in brain-wave patterns (showing less excitability), and that it strengthens the immune system and endocrine system (hormones).

The unusual thing about meditation is that it involves 'letting go', allowing the mind to roam freely. Most of us are used to trying to control our thoughts – in our work, for example – so letting go is not as easy as it sounds.

It may help to know that people who regularly meditate say they have more energy, require less sleep, are less anxious, and feel 'more alive' than they did before. Ideally, the technique should be taught by a skilled instructor – but as meditation is essentially performed alone it can be learned alone with equal success.

Meditation may sound a bit off-beat to you. But isn't it worth a try – especially when you can do it for free? Kick off those shoes and make yourself comfortable somewhere you can be alone for a while. Now follow these simple instructions:

1 Close your eyes, relax, and practise the deep-breathing exercise as described above.
2 Concentrate on your breathing. Try to free your mind of conscious control.

3 Letting your mind roam unchecked, try to allow the deeper, more serene part of you to take over.
4 If you wish to go further into meditation, concentrate on mentally repeating a 'mantra' – a certain word or short phrase. It should be something positive, such as 'Relax', 'I feel calm', or even 'I am special'.
5 When you are ready to finish, open your eyes and allow yourself time to adjust to the outside world before getting to your feet.

The aim of mentally repeating a mantra is to plant positive thoughts into your subconscious mind. It is a form of self-hypnosis; you alone control the messages placed there.

When to seek medical help

Self-treatment cannot always keep hay fever symptoms under control. You should seek medical help as soon as possible in any of these circumstances:

- when self-treatment fails to provide symptom relief;
- if a sore throat gets progressively worse instead of better;
- if your nasal secretions become coloured, thick or bloody – they should be clear.

If you experience serious symptoms, such as any of the following, go immediately to the emergency department of your local hospital:

- prolonged feverishness
- a very high temperature
- difficulty breathing
- uncontrolled bleeding from the nose
- severe earache or a discharge from the ear.

7

A nutritional approach

Hay fever is a disorder in which the balance of the body is affected – caused largely by adrenal exhaustion and a hypersensitized immune system. These vital systems should, therefore, be supported by working from every angle possible to help the body back into balance. When bodily systems are strengthened and once again networking properly, the errors will begin to correct themselves. A vital area of support is improved nutrition, for among its many benefits, it is of enormous help to the body at the important cellular level.

Cell health

The human body is capable of complete rejuvenation, regeneration and repair. In other words, it can heal itself, given the right conditions, mentally and physically. Good nutrition is the most vital factor towards good physical health, for it allows our cells – the smallest but most important components in our bodies – to be nourished continually and washed clean of waste. Our cells do not function at optimum levels if they are seldom fed and cleansed. In fact, poor nutrition diminishes cell function, causes gradual toxic build-up within the cells, triggers disease and exacerbates the ageing process.

Although we have much to eat in Western societies, our food has frighteningly little nutritional value, having been grown in overused soils that are loaded with harmful chemicals and lacking in essential minerals. Needing a boost of energy and a feeling of sustenance, we turn to stimulants such as coffee, sugar, junk food and alcohol. However, these are actually toxic substances, which make the liver hyperactive in its attempt to filter out the toxins, and which weaken the adrenal glands. This, in turn, speeds up the metabolism, which demands a short yet intense energy capacity that is stolen from the cells and the immune system. As a result, the body feels fatigued – and the longer the cycle of harmful diet continues, the more fatigued the body becomes, at the cellular level.

This situation – called acidosis – is reflected in the individual's mental, physical and emotional make-up. It creates a seriously ineffective immune system and a body that is struggling to run on empty. The acidosis causes imbalances within the organs, the digestive tract and the cells, allowing parasites, unfriendly bacteria, fungi and viruses to take over and normally innocuous substances to be seen as allergenic.

Our cells are being replaced constantly on a rotational basis. With the correct help (see below) each unhealthy old cell can be replaced by a healthy new one, leading to better health in totality. However, this takes time. Imagine a neglected houseplant which you then start feeding and watering appropriately. The leaves perk up a bit from the improved nutrition, but you have to wait for the old leaves to die off and the new ones to grow before you are left with a truly healthy plant. It is the same with the human body. When you start feeding and treating it better, you have to wait for the physiological dynamics of the body to produce new improved cells in every area.

How it used to be

There has been little change to our bodies, in a genetic or physiological sense, since the days of the ancient hunter-gatherer. Our basic foodstuffs are very similar too. What has changed, and dramatically, is our lifestyle, behaviour and diet – the latter having altered a great deal in just the last 50–60 years. Nature takes a long time to make changes, whereas humans can make radical shifts within a generation or two. This is much too fast to expect our bodies to adjust.

Our diet today consists largely of processed foods – that is, food grown on land laden with chemicals, which has been altered in some way by human hand, and which also contains chemical preservatives, flavourings and colourings. We generally consume our foods in a rushed and stressful environment too – eating, reading or working at the same time; whereas in ancient times people would usually just concentrate on eating. Their foods were not sprayed with chemicals or injected with preservatives, they were eaten fresh and in season – and fresh, uncontaminated fruit and vegetables are highly nutritious. They are also rich in enzymes, the substances that aid digestion. For the most part, our forebears' food was uncooked. Both cooking (above 41°C/107°F) and refrigeration destroy live digestive enzymes, which help break down the food in our bodies.

Because our ancestors consumed freshly gathered, uncontaminated 'whole' foods, their digestive systems would have functioned superbly, with the added benefit of fresh air and exercise contributing to their good health. It is doubtful that ancient humans developed hay fever.

However, hay fever is a condition that can improve considerably if we can get back to basics, diet-wise.

The aim of a hay fever diet

As mentioned above, the average Western diet is nowadays very poor. It is estimated that we eat approximately 17 per cent of our daily calories as processed foods, 18 per cent as saturated fats, 18 per cent as sugar and 3 to 10 per cent as alcoholic beverages. When you add this up, more than half of our foods are high in calories and low in nutrients. So it is little wonder that over time many of us develop chronic health problems.

Eating a lot of refined carbohydrates, junk foods, additives and so on can cause stress to the adrenal glands, which eventually weakens them – and weakened adrenal glands are capable of producing a multitude of symptoms and disorders, which can include the inflammatory response that characterizes hay fever. However, if you already suffer from hay fever, your adrenal glands must be weakened already. It is advisable, therefore, that you do all you can to prevent their function from deteriorating further. The advice in this book should help you to undo the harm and add strength to the adrenal glands and immune system.

In brief, a diet tailored for hay fever sufferers focuses on helping you to do the following:

- Reduce mucus-forming foods that may stimulate the excessive production of catarrh. Such foods include dairy, wheat, gluten and sugars (see below).
- Reduce consumption of foods to which your body is sensitive and which may either cause additional reactions or worsen an existing allergy reaction (see page 27 for information on oral allergy syndrome).
- Reduce your intake of toxins, particularly the colourings, flavourings and preservatives contained in most processed, prepackaged foods. They cause problems in many bodily systems.
- Reduce your consumption of stimulants which, among other things, cause stress to the adrenal glands.
- Eat a low-acid diet, to reduce acidosis in the body.
- Eat more organic 'wholefoods' (see below).
- Increase your intake of vitamin C, which can strengthen the immune system. In addition, the adrenal cortex requires a lot of

vitamin C to synthesize the hormones it produces (see pages 89–90 for more information on vitamin C).

- Take supplements to boost your nutritional intake (see below).

It's also worth noting that changing over to healthy eating, which this diet basically is, can help to counter the depression and fatigue experienced by many people with hay fever.

A 'wholefood' diet

Wholefoods are simply those that have had nothing taken away (nutrients and fibre, for example) and that have had nothing added (in the form of colourings, flavourings or preservatives). In short, they are foods in their most natural form. Wholefoods that are organically produced – without the use of potentially dangerous chemical fertilizers, pesticides and herbicides – are even better for us.

If a streaming nose and watery eyes mean that you find it difficult to think about cooking in the conventional way, a range of organic convenience foods using wholefood ingredients is now available from health food shops and some supermarkets. You could try these, perhaps, until you are feeling more able to get back to normal.

Fresh vegetables

Fresh vegetables not only have alkalizing properties, they are rich in vitamin C and other important vitamins and minerals. It is therefore recommended that you try to eat as many as you can, selecting locally grown, organic vegetables that are in season – these have the highest nutrient content and the greatest enzyme activity. Enzymes are to our body what spark plugs are to the car engine. Without its 'sparks', the body doesn't work properly. Organically grown vegetables may not look as perfect as those that are processed, but they *are* superior – processed foods are devitalized of their 'sparks'. Try to eat as fresh and as raw as possible; make a variety of salads and aim to eat one every day. When you do cook vegetables, use as little water as possible (preferably unsalted, or only lightly), and cook for the minimum length of time. Lightly steaming and stir-frying are healthy alternatives. Scrub rather than peel your vegetables.

Legumes (peas and beans)

Legumes contain high amounts of protein, and they are inexpensive. The soya bean is a complete protein, and there are many soya bean products, including soya milk, tofu, tempeh and miso. Tofu is very versatile and can be used in both savoury and sweet dishes. Soya milk can be used as an alternative to cow's milk, which due to its mucus-forming components, is not recommended in hay fever (see below).

Seeds

Seeds – sunflower, sesame, hemp, flax and pumpkin, for example – contain a wonderful combination of the nutrients necessary to start a new plant, and are very important to strengthening the immune system. They can be eaten as they come as a snack, sprinkled on to salads and cereals, or used in baking. For more flavour they can be lightly roasted and coated with organic soy sauce. Cracked linseed and pumpkin seeds are highly nutritious and useful for treating constipation. They can be used in baking and sprinkled on to breakfast cereals, over salads, in soups and added to porridge oats.

Nuts

Nuts, too, are an intrinsic part of strengthening the immune system. All nuts contain vital nutrients, but almonds, cashews, walnuts, brazils and pecans perhaps offer the greatest array. Eat a wide assortment as snacks, with breakfast cereal and in baking.

As peanuts are capable of provoking violent life-threatening allergic reactions in some people, you may wish to avoid nuts completely. However, many hay fever sufferers never experience adverse reactions to nuts of any kind. They are a valuable addition to your diet, but whether or not you eat nuts is entirely up to you – and it is just as well to be cautious.

Grains

Wholegrains and wholemeal flours provide the complex unrefined carbohydrates that our bodies require – and again organic is best. Many types of grain are good for us, but wheat – our staple in the West – contains gluten and can be highly allergenic, so should be avoided. Barring wheat, aim to consume a variety of grains, including oats, rye, barley (generally available as pearl barley), corn, buckwheat, brown rice and mixed grains. Brown rice, millet, buckwheat and maize/corn are all gluten-free and invaluable to people with a gluten allergy/sensitivity.

Fats and oils

Fats (fatty acids) are the most concentrated sources of energy in our diet; 1 gram of fat provides the body with nine calories of energy. They are also a good source of vitamin E, which is a natural antihistamine. There are two distinct types of fat, *saturated* and *unsaturated*.

Saturated fat is believed to be implicated in the development of heart disease, and comes mainly from animal sources. It is generally solid at room temperature. Although for many years margarine was believed to be a healthier choice over butter, nutritionists have now revised their opinion; some of the fats in the margarine hydrogenation process are changed into trans-fatty acids, which the body metabolizes as if they were saturated fatty acids – the same as butter. Butter is a valuable source of oils and vitamin A, but should be used very sparingly. Margarine, on the other hand, is an artificial product containing many additives, and not recommended in hay fever.

Unsaturated fat, also called polyunsaturated or monounsaturated fat, has a protective effect on the heart and other organs. Omega-3 and omega-6 oils occur naturally in oily fish (mackerel, herring, sardines, tuna), nuts and seeds, and is usually liquid at room temperature. It is recommended that people with hay fever eat oily fish at least three times a week and use cold-pressed oil (olive, rapeseed, safflower and sunflower oil) daily, in salad dressings and cooking.

Eggs

You're no doubt aware that eggs are high in cholesterol, which is a type of fat. However, they also contain lecithin, which is a superb biological detergent capable of breaking down fats so they can be utilized by the body. Lecithin also prevents the accumulation of too many acid or alkaline substances in the blood and encourages the transport of nutrients through the cell walls. Eggs should be soft-boiled or poached as a hard yolk will bind the lecithin, rendering it useless as a fat detergent. Try to eat two or three eggs a week.

Garlic

Eating garlic on a regular basis can help to reduce excess mucus production. It is recommended that, if possible, people with hay fever eat two raw cloves a day – perhaps on toast or stirred into food in the latter stages of cooking. If you really can't bear to eat your garlic raw, or don't like garlic at all, try taking a garlic supplement, available from most supermarkets, health food shops and chemists.

Fish

Try to increase your intake of omega-3 fatty acids by eating plenty of cold-water fish, especially oily fish such as sardines, fresh tuna, anchovies, mackerel, trout, salmon, herring (kippers) and pilchards. Such fish also provide gamma linoleic acid (GLA), a deficiency of which can encourage inflammation and so aggravate allergic conditions. GLA deficiency is often evident as dry skin, premenstrual syndrome (PMS) in women and sometimes eczema.

For maximum benefit, try to avoid frying your fish or covering it in breadcrumbs.

Sprouted foods

When foods are sprouted, dormant enzymes spring into action, providing more nutrients per gram than any other natural food. They can therefore help to normalize all the body's systems, including the immune system which is weakened and hypersensitive in hay fever. A mixture of different sprouts is capable even of supporting life all on their own – although this is not recommended! Sprouted foods are also very inexpensive. You could try sprouting seeds and beans yourself so that you have your own supply.

Fresh seeds, beans and grains will sprout when rinsed and placed in pure water in a plastic bowl or polythene bag. The container should be sealed and placed in an airing cupboard or by a radiator for three to four days, changing the liquid twice a day. A dose of light and sunshine will make them ready for eating. Eat your sprouted foods in salads and soups.

Be aware, however, that seed potatoes and tomatoes should not be sprouted – they belong to the deadly nightshade family. Kidney bean sprouts are poisonous too.

Yogurt

Yogurt can slightly reduce the amount of histamine produced during an allergic reaction. It also helps to cool and soothe a sore throat. For hay fever, eat plain (unflavoured) organic acidophilus yogurt – one or two tubs a day, if possible. It is particularly useful to use this kind of yogurt after taking a course of antibiotics (see pages 37–8). Organic acidophilus yogurt is available from most health food shops and some supermarkets.

Wheat

Although wheat is the staple grain in Western societies, its gluten content is often identified as an allergen by a hypersensitive immune system. If you are allergic to the gluten in wheat, you are likely to experience a streaming nose and other symptoms that are reminiscent of hay fever, as well as possibly asthma and itchiness in the scalp, skin and throat. If you are unsure whether you are allergic to wheat, follow the food elimination programme described in Chapter 3 to see if your symptoms improve.

Many people with hay fever have a reaction to wheat and find that eliminating it from their diet and replacing it with oats, rye, barley, corn, buckwheat, brown rice and mixed grains helps to alleviate their symptoms.

Oats

Mentioned briefly above, oats warrant further attention here as they have many benefits. They provide a slow release of energy, which helps to stabilize blood sugar levels; they also nourish the central nervous system and are rich in minerals and the B vitamins. Therefore they help the body to normalize itself and reduce its overreaction to normal environmental substances, such as pollen. Try to eat a bowl of porridge for breakfast every day, and buy oatmeal biscuits and oat cereal bars.

Foods to reduce or eliminate

It is known that reducing or eliminating certain foods can improve hay fever symptoms.

Reduce omega-6, increase omega-3

In Western societies our dietary habits are believed to have contributed to the increase in hay fever during the last decade or so. This is, to some extent, because we tend to consume proportionately larger amounts of omega-6 fatty acids, in the form of meat and dairy products, than omega-3 fatty acids which are present in foods such as fish, nuts and seeds. Indeed, a range of studies have strongly indicated that eating a higher percentage of omega-6 than omega-3 fatty acids can actually worsen allergy symptoms. It therefore makes sense that consuming more foods containing omega-3 fatty acids will have a protective effect, reducing symptoms, while the reverse is likely to be the case with omega-6 fatty acids.

Excellent omega-3 fatty acid sources include flaxseeds, salmon, cabbage, fresh mustard seed, cauliflower, scallops, walnuts, ground cloves, ground oregano and baked and infused peppermint leaves. Other good sources include Brussels sprouts, lettuce, French beans, broccoli, turnip, collard greens, strawberries, tofu, soya beans, halibut, shrimp, snapper, cod, tuna and yellowfin.

Dairy produce

Dairy products contain omega-6 fatty acids, which are believed to worsen allergy symptoms; they also promote the formation of mucus and can encourage inflammation. Cutting out dairy altogether would probably significantly benefit your hay fever, but it is not recommended as the calcium in dairy foods is essential for building and maintaining strong bones and teeth. Children, pregnant and breastfeeding women, and people with the bone-thinning disease osteoporosis need substantial amounts of dairy produce; however, other groups can manage very well by cutting out cow's milk products and replacing them with milk products from goats and sheep. There is also soya milk and rice milk, which provide many nutrients.

Unless you belong to one of the groups mentioned above, try to limit your consumption of animal milk products or cut them out altogether.

Red meat

As mentioned above, red meat contains omega-6 fatty acids, which it is thought worsen allergy symptoms. And like dairy produce, red meat is mucus-forming, so all in all it is not the best food for someone with hay fever. It doesn't help either that animals are generally reared with the use of hormones, antibiotics and pesticides, which are especially detrimental in allergy conditions. It is recommended, therefore, that you try to cut down on red meat as much as possible. If you do eat red meat, make sure that it is organic (free from hormones, antibiotics and pesticides) and the portion size is no larger or thicker than the palm of your hand. Try to eat alternative sources of protein such as goat's cheese, beans, pulses and soya products.

Carbohydrates

The adrenal cortex (the outer section of the adrenal gland) is very sensitive to simple (refined) carbohydrates and may, after repeated intake, set up an inflammatory response. Indeed, consumption of these 'bad carb' foods – pastries, cakes, sweets, sweetened fruit juice, refined and unrefined sugar, and biscuits – is believed by some experts to give rise to allergic disease such as hay fever. Cut down on these simple carbohydrates as much as possible, trying even to eliminate them completely during an allergic attack. Doing so can greatly reduce your symptoms.

Consumption of complex carbohydrates – commonly known as the 'good carbs' and including vegetables, breads, cereal, legumes and pasta – is recommended in hay fever.

Fruit

Try to avoid eating too much fruit, especially oranges. Although rich in vitamin C and many other nutrients, fruits are also full of sugar which is a mucus-forming food. You can still obtain large amounts of vitamin C by eating fresh vegetables and the other foods recommended earlier in this chapter, and you should boost your intake with supplements of vitamin C, as recommended below.

Cigarettes and alcohol

One of the main reasons that human beings crave stimulants such as cigarettes and alcohol, and also caffeine and products containing refined white sugar (see below), is high levels of stress. When, for example, hay fever symptoms are making you feel stressed, your body demands a boost – a 'lift'. However, the lift obtained from cigarettes and alcohol is short-lived – unlike the damage it can do to your adrenal glands, which are already tired and weakened in hay fever. Stimulants can create a hypersensitive immune system, chronic anxiety, low energy, nerve cell damage and much more. Moreover, stimulants of any kind are known to aggravate allergy symptoms.

If you find you are unable to completely eliminate stimulants from your life, reduce them as much as possible – it *will* make a difference.

Sugar

Sugar is, as already mentioned, a mucus-forming food, but its consumption has also been linked with a number of disorders from diabetes to heart disease and cancer. We do need a certain amount of sugar in our diet, which we can get naturally from foods such as fruits (see above) and complex carbohydrates for conversion to energy. Don't worry, however, that if you cut down on the amount of fruit you eat (as recommended in hay fever) you won't be getting the natural sugar that you need. Following the hay fever diet as described in this book will ensure that you get enough.

If you must add sweetening to your food and drinks, alternatives to refined white sugar include raw honey and barley malt. Although sugar is best avoided (as highlighted on page 84), muscovado (which is referred to as 'soft brown sugar') and Demerara sugars are formed during the early stages of the sugar refining process and so contain more nutrients than refined white sugar. All these alternatives may be used in cooking and baking.

You may be wondering whether refined white sugar can be replaced by a sugar substitute such as aspartame, sold under the brand names of NutraSweet, Spoonful, Equal and Indulge. Well, the short answer, if you really want to be healthy, is no. Aspartame is an excitatory neuro-transmitter that causes nerve cells to fire continually until they become exhausted and die. Many people consume food and drinks containing aspartame in an attempt to lose weight. However, it creates a craving for simple carbohydrates, which only gives rise to an increase in weight. When the person stops ingesting aspartame – in diet drinks, for example – he or she generally loses weight. Fortunately, there are natural sweeteners such as Stevia and Xylitol that are perfectly safe and these are available from health food shops.

Caffeine

Caffeine products – which include coffee, tea, cocoa, cola drinks and chocolate – cause stress to the adrenal glands, which make it difficult for the body to cope with stress. The adrenal glands are tired and weakened anyway in hay fever, so continuing to use stimulants of any kind can only make the situation worse. Caffeine products are also toxic to the liver, detrimental to the nervous system and can reduce the body's ability to absorb vitamins and minerals. Consumed regularly in fairly high doses, caffeine is likely to give rise to chronic anxiety, the symptoms of which are agitation, palpitations, headaches, indigestion, panic, insomnia and hyperventilation. My best advice is to remove caffeine products from your diet.

The addictiveness of caffeine makes reduction far from easy, however, and withdrawal symptoms can take the form of splitting headaches, fatigue, depression, poor concentration and muscle pains. It's no wonder people can feel terrible until they have had their first dose of caffeine in the morning, and that they can't seem to function properly without regular doses throughout the day! Fortunately, caffeine is quickly 'washed out' of the system, and it is possible to minimize withdrawal symptoms by reducing your intake over several weeks.

A problem can be finding an acceptable alternative. Coffee, tea, cocoa and cola drinks can be replaced by fruit juices (limited intake only), vegetable juices and herbal teas (green tea is very good; as is rooibosch (redbush) tea); the latter two are low in tannin and high in antioxidants. A variety of grain coffee substitutes may also be purchased from health food shops. As many decaffeinated products are processed with the use of chemicals, they are, unfortunately, not a good choice.

Carob, which is similar to the cocoa bean, is a healthy, caffeine-free alternative to cocoa and chocolate. It contains less fat and is naturally sweet, unlike the cocoa bean which is bitter and needs sweetening. Carob bars can therefore be an enjoyable replacement for chocolate bars and other confectionery. Carob is also available in powder form for use in baking and in drinks.

Salt

Due to its ability to inhibit the growth of harmful micro-organisms, high levels of salt are added as a preservative to most processed and prepackaged foods. For example, one tin of soup can contain more salt (sodium) than the recommended daily allowance for an adult. Large amounts of salt are also added to most breakfast cereals, except for shredded wheat products. You can limit your intake of salt by reducing your consumption of processed and prepackaged foods, or buying only those labelled 'low salt' or 'sodium free'. In baking and cooking, use only a very small amount of sea salt or rock salt, and try to avoid sprinkling any type of salt over your meals. Reducing your salt intake very gradually is the best way to retrain your palate.

Artificial colourings

Today's processed foods often contain artificial colourings, such as tartrazine, to make them more appealing to the consumer. However, food colourings are derived from petroleum and contain toxic compounds that have been linked to many diseases. If you can't avoid buying processed foods, read the list of ingredients carefully to ensure that there are no artificial colourings. It's always best to buy fresh foods, however.

Useful vitamins and minerals

The vitamins and minerals recommended in the treatment of hay fever should be taken in combination for approximately three months before your symptoms generally begin.

It's important to note that in most instances, the recommended daily allowances (RDAs) of vitamin and mineral supplements, set by the Department of Health, are only intended to prevent common diseases associated with a severe deficiency. They do not indicate amounts that promote the optimal functioning and protection of bodily systems. RDAs are, therefore, the very *minimum* intake for good health. For example, the RDA for vitamin E is 10 mg, but scientific research has shown that the level offering protection to the heart is in excess of 67 mg. Of course, this amount includes the vitamin E obtained from natural sources.

Vitamin A (beta carotene)

Intake of sufficient vitamin A (in the form of beta carotene) is vital to the good health of all the bodily tissues – it also reduces inflammation and promotes good health of the mucous membranes throughout the respiratory tract. Therefore, in hay fever, greater than average amounts of this nutrient are required on a daily basis. Beta carotene food sources include yellow and orange vegetables and fruits (but limit your intake of fruits) such as carrots, sweet potatoes, apricot, cantaloupe, papaya, pumpkin, melon and mango. This compound can also be found in dark, leafy vegetables such as spinach, Brussels sprouts, broccoli, watercress, cabbage and parsley. Due to their high mineral content, seaweeds such as kelp, nori, kombu and wakame are useful too.

Vitamin A (beta carotene) supplementation – that is, taken in tablet or capsule form – can also be helpful in the treatment of hay fever, the recommended daily dosage being 25,000 IUs (International Units). This supplement should not be taken during pregnancy, however.

When vitamin A (beta carotene) is taken in conjunction with vitamin E as a preventative measure, there can be a significant impact on hay fever symptoms. Vitamin A (beta carotene) taken in combination with vitamin C (bioflavonoids) for three months before the hay fever season commences can also make a difference.

B-complex vitamins

All the B vitamins are invaluable for the reduction of stress, regulation of the nervous system and production of energy. They can also help to normalize the immune system so that it is less likely to identify innocuous substances as allergenic. Unlike most other vitamins, the B vitamins are all interdependent, meaning they work best when in combination with each other.

B vitamins can be obtained from wholegrains, lentils, seeds, leafy green vegetables, oily fish, avocados, prunes, apricots, mushrooms, dried fruit, eggs, lean meat and poultry. However, the B vitamins tend to be unstable, which makes them easily destroyed in food preparation and cooking. Furthermore, they are quickly flushed through the body, so need to be replenished on a daily basis. One daily comprehensive supplement tablet can be of great benefit, especially if your hay fever symptoms are making you feel stressed. Follow the label dosage instructions.

Vitamin B5 (pantothenic acid)

This nutrient is intimately involved in the immune response, which would indicate that boosting its levels in your body can aid in normalizing the immune system. It can also help to combat adrenal exhaustion. If your symptoms are severe, take 250 mg three times daily between meals for a few days – in addition to a B-complex supplement – reducing the dose to 100 mg, three times daily, for up to a month.

Vitamin B12

As vitamin B12 works to reduce the inflammatory response, it can be of great benefit in hay fever. B12 is only found in animal products, although as stated above beef products and dairy products from cow's milk are not recommended in those with allergies, and some people dislike products from alternatives such as goats and sheep. However, B12 is present in poultry and fish, so try to use these as your source. Vitamin B12 supplementation is recommended at 1,000 mcg daily, taken in the morning.

Vitamin C and bioflavonoids

Vitamin C is an important nutrient that is required in higher quantities than normal in hay fever. This is because the adrenal cortex uses vitamin C to synthesize the hormones it produces, as discussed in Chapter 4. Several studies into the effect of high doses of vitamin C on hay fever symptoms have shown that it has properties similar to many antihistamines, but without the side effects. Unfortunately, vitamin C is quickly used up in the body, especially by smoking, alcohol consumption, surgery, trauma, stress, exposure to pollutants and the use of certain medications. Fruits – a rich source of vitamin C – are mucus-forming foods so should be eaten in moderation; however, there are some exceptions, such as strawberries, blueberries (bilberries) and raspberries, which are high in bioflavonoids (see below). Other hay fever-friendly food sources are broccoli, Brussels sprouts, cabbage, sauerkraut, cauliflower, kale, turnips, spinach, potatoes and peppers (capsicum). As this vitamin is easily destroyed by heat and overprocessing, cook your vegetables, preferably by steaming, for as little time as possible.

It is highly recommended to use vitamin C supplementation as part of your treatment regime. Look for the type that is combined with bio-flavonoids, such as quercetin, catechin and hesperidin – these compounds have an anti-inflammatory effect on the mucous membranes. Bioflavonoids also increase the effectiveness of vitamin C by preventing it from being depleted by smoking, alcohol consumption and so on. In effect, bioflavonoids are able to greatly improve the body's ability to absorb and retain vitamin C. In the treatment of hay fever, it is recommended that you take 1,000 mg three to five times a day.

Vitamin E

One of the main benefits of vitamin E in the treatment of hay fever is its natural antihistamine properties. It is also important for maintaining a good oxygen supply to the nerve cells and protecting red blood cells from toxins. In a range of studies, volunteers who consumed large amounts of EPA (see below) and vitamin E were found to have a lower than average risk of developing hay fever. Note, however, that vitamin E has anti-coagulant properties, so anyone taking drugs such as warfarin and heparin should consult their doctor before supplementing their vitamin E intake.

In hay fever, good vitamin E food sources are fish, egg yolks, leafy green vegetables, and oil, seed and grain derivatives, including wheat-germ, safflower, avocados, nuts, sunflower oil and seeds, pumpkin seeds, linseeds, almonds, brazils, cashews, pecans, wholegrain cereals and breads, wheatgerm, asparagus, dried prunes and broccoli. Be careful with oil-containing foods, however, which should be kept in an airtight container away from sunlight: rancid oils are extremely damaging to the body.

Supplements of vitamin E are widely available from supermarkets and chemists. It is recommended that people with hay fever take 400 IUs on a daily basis, starting three months before the hay fever season commences.

Selenium

This important trace mineral protects cells from the toxic effects of harmful free radicals in the body, and so can help to normalize the immune system. Hay fever-friendly food sources include tuna, salmon, shrimp, garlic, tomatoes, brazil nuts, turkey, chicken, duck, rice, walnuts, cottage cheese, macaroni, noodles, spaghetti and sunflower seeds. If you wish to take this mineral in supplement form, the RDA for hay fever is 100 mcg.

Zinc

Zinc is involved in a wide range of metabolic activities and is required for good functioning of the immune system. People with hay fever are often deficient in zinc. Good zinc food sources include the herb liquorice, seafood, (lean) meats, eggs, liver, wheatgerm, pumpkin seeds, sunflower seeds and ginseng. If you take zinc in supplement form, follow the label dosage instructions.

Co-Enzyme Q10

Also known as CoQ10, this enzyme is an important aid to people with hay fever as it benefits the immune system, reduces the allergic response and helps to alleviate fatigue. A powerful antioxidant, it works by aiding the transfer of oxygen and energy between components of the cells and between the blood and the tissues. Good food sources are mackerel, nuts, chicken, wholegrains, wild salmon, sardines and spinach. CoQ10 can be purchased in capsule form from most health food shops.

8

Complementary therapies

Increasing numbers of people with allergies are turning to complementary therapies, such as acupuncture and aromatherapy, often using them in conjunction with their conventional allergy medication. If you are using or thinking about trying complementary therapies, please be aware that some can cause adverse reactions in certain people, and the quality and strength of treatments are not controlled by a regulating body. In comparison with mainstream medicine which is supported by a great deal of research, very few studies and/or controlled scientific trials into the effects of complementary medicine have been carried out. Before deciding to use a particular therapy, try to find out as much about it as you can. You could also ask your doctor's advice.

That said, people with hay fever often report a significant benefit from using complementary therapies, although this may partly stem from knowing they are doing something positive to help themselves. There is no doubt that the more relaxing therapies can reduce the stress caused by the symptoms of hay fever.

Acupuncture

An ancient form of oriental healing, acupuncture involves puncturing the skin with fine needles at specific points in the body. These points are located along energy channels (meridians) that are believed to be blocked where allergy is present. This energy is known as chi (also spelt qi). Needles are inserted to increase, decrease or unblock the flow of chi energy so that the balance of yin and yang is restored.

Yin, the female force, is calm and passive; it also represents dark, cold, swelling and moisture. On the other hand, yang, the male force, is stimulating and aggressive, representing heat, light, contraction and dryness. It is thought that an imbalance in these forces is the cause of illness and disease. For example, a person who feels the cold, and suffers fluid retention and fatigue, would be considered to have an excess of yin. A person experiencing repeated headaches, however, will be deemed to have an excess of yang. Emotional, physical or environmental factors are believed to disturb the chi energy balance, and can also be treated. I should mention here that according to acupuncturists, following a healthy balanced diet, as recommended in Chapter 7, can go a long way towards restoring the balance of yin and yang.

In your acupuncture session, the therapist determines your particular acupuncture points – it is thought there are as many as 2,000 points on the body and a set method is used to establish where exactly they are. At a consultation, questions may be asked about your lifestyle, sleeping patterns, fears, phobias and reactions to stress. Your pulses will be felt, after which the acupuncture itself is carried out, very fine needles being placed at the relevant sites. The first consultation will normally last for an hour, and you should notice a change for the better after four to six sessions.

Acupuncturists report that they can improve hay fever by treating points along the meridians that correspond to the areas that produce the worst hay fever symptoms. Unblocking the energy channels causes symptoms to decline and even to disappear. Such treatments are claimed also to support adrenal function and regulate the immune system, stopping it from reacting to inoffensive substances as if they were harmful. Acupuncturists say that they achieve higher success rates if the treatment is begun a few weeks prior to the hay fever season, rather than during it.

Acupuncture is undoubtedly a very safe therapy. The only very slight risk is that of infection from the needles.

Aromatherapy

Certain health disorders can be helped by the use of aromatic oils – known as essential oils. It is believed that stimulating our sense of smell with a particular aroma can help to treat a particular health problem. There's no doubt at all that aromatherapy can aid relaxation and help to reduce the anxiety, tension and irritability often associated with hay fever.

Concentrated essential oils are extracted from plants and may either be inhaled, rubbed directly into the skin or used in bathing. Each odour relates to its plant of origin, being a concentrated version of the aroma of the original plant, such as lavender or geranium.

Plant essences have been used for healing throughout the ages, and smaller amounts are used for aromatherapy purposes than in herbal medicines. Aromatherapy oils are obtained either by steaming a particular plant extract until the oil glands burst, or by soaking the plant extract in hot oil so that the cells collapse and release their essence.

Techniques used in aromatherapy

These are the main methods used in aromatherapy:

- *Inhalation* – Giving the fastest result, the inhalation of essential oils has a direct influence on the olfactory (nasal) organs, and is immediately received by the brain. Steam inhalation is the most popular technique. Mix a few drops of oil with a bowlful of boiling water and lean over it to breathe in the steam, or use an oil burner, whereby the flame from a tealight candle heats a small saucer of water containing a few drops of oil.
- *Massage* – Essential oils intended for massage are normally prediluted. They should never be applied to the skin in an undilute (pure) form. When using undiluted essential oils, mix three or four drops with a neutral carrier oil such as olive or safflower oil. The oils penetrate the skin, and are absorbed by the body, and this is believed to exert a positive influence on a particular organ or set of tissues.
- *Bathing* – Tension and anxiety can be reduced by using aromatherapy oils in the bath. A few drops of pure essential oil should be added directly to running tap water – it mixes more efficiently this way. No more than 20 drops of oil in total should be used.

Oils for treating hay fever

The following essential oils are believed to have beneficial effects:

- *Tea tree* (contains terpenes, alcoloids and cineol) – Reputed to purify the respiratory system, relieve sinus infections, stimulate elimination through the throat and lungs and strengthen breathing. As an expectorant, it stimulates and liquefies mucus production to ease nasal and sinus congestion.
- *Rosemary* (contains cineol, alcoloids, esters and ketones) – Cleanses the lymphatic system, eases respiratory conditions and stimulates elimination through the lungs.
- *Sandalwood* (contains santolol) – Stimulates mucus secretions to ease nasal and lung congestion. It can also help to combat fatigue.

Terpenes work to drain and dry mucus; alcoloids work to energize and can help to combat infections; cineol works as an expectorant to loosen bronchial mucus; ketones work to dissolve thick mucus and aid respiratory problems; santolol works to clean the lymphatic system and aid respiratory problems.

Using a blend of oils

A blend of the above-mentioned oils can reduce the symptoms of hay fever, calm the respiratory system, reduce itchiness and irritation in the mucous membranes and dry much of the nasal discharge. Use them together in the following combinations:

- *For massage* – Place three drops of each of the three essential oils above in a bowl with 25 drops of a neutral carrier oil such as olive or safflower oil. Mix together and use for a gentle massage in the upper back and chest areas.
- *For inhalation* – Place one drop of one or more of the three above oils in a bowl of boiling water and inhale. Lean over the bowl and cover your head and the bowl with a towel to prevent the fumes escaping.

Oils for relaxation

Lavender is the most popular oil for relaxation. It is known to be a wonderful restorative and excellent for relieving tension headaches as well as stress. Other oils that can be used alone or blended to provide a relaxing atmosphere include Roman camomile and ylang ylang. Ylang ylang has relaxing properties, including a calming effect on the heart-rate, and can relieve palpitations and raised blood pressure. Camomile can be very soothing too, and aids both sleep and digestion.

Drop your relaxation oils into the vessel part of an oil burner and top up with water. Light a tealight candle beneath the burner and relax while the essential oils scent the whole room and you inhale their fragrance. Such oils are safe around babies and children, as rather than being overpowering the aroma is soft and soothing.

Try one of the following combinations. In each case, blend the oils well and diffuse in a burner. The first two combinations can also be added to 2 fl oz of distilled water, shaken well and used in a spray bottle for a non-toxic room freshener with relaxing properties.

- 5 drops lavender, 2 drops Roman camomile and 1 drop ylang ylang.
- 8 drops mandarin, 3 drops neroli and 3 drops ylang ylang.
- 10 drops bergamot, 2 drops rose otto and 3 drops Roman camomile.

For relaxation, this is a great blend for use in the bath:

- 3 drops lavender, 2 drops marjoram, 2 drops basil, 1 drop vetiver, 1 drop fennel.

Hypnotherapy

Hypnotherapy has been described as psychotherapy using hypnosis. There is, however, still no acceptable definition of the actual state of hypnosis. It is commonly described as an altered state of consciousness, lying somewhere between being awake and being asleep. People under hypnosis are aware of their surroundings, yet their minds are to a large extent under the control of the hypnotist. Subjects also seem to pass control of their actions, as well as a chunk of their thoughts, to the hypnotist. We have all seen people under hypnosis on TV, acting out a role. At the time they are absorbed in what they have been 'told' to do – often instigated by a specific 'trigger' word – but immediately afterwards they wonder what on earth they were doing. It's clear that their behaviour has been dictated, to a certain extent, by the hypnotist. Hypno*therapy*, however, is about the hypnotist using the power of hypnotism for therapeutic purposes.

Hypnotherapy is performed by putting the patient into a 'trance' state. You may have heard that in the early nineteenth century some surgeons actually used hypnotism – then called 'mesmerism' – to perform pain-free operations. At the time, however, the majority of the medical profession were highly sceptical of this practice, believing that patients had been schooled or paid to show no pain. It is only in the last two decades that hypnotism has become an accepted form of therapy.

Nowadays, a hypnotherapist will take a full psychological and physiological history of each patient before slowly talking them into a trance state. The therapist can use either direct suggestion – intimating that the patient's symptoms will notably lessen – or will begin to explore the root cause of any tension, anxiety or depression. Of course, the exact nature of the therapy depends largely on the problem for which treatment is being sought.

One common fear is that the therapist may, while the patient is in a trance, implant dangerous suggestions or extract improper personal information. However, I would stress that patients can come out of a trance at any time, particularly if they are asked to do or say anything they would not contemplate when awake. And malpractice would only have to be brought to light once to ruin the therapist's career. You may prefer to visit a hypnotherapist recommended by your doctor.

Some hypnotherapy experts believe that the main purpose of hypnotherapy is to promote relaxation, reduce tension, increase confidence and make a person more able to cope with problems. However, there has been at least one study into the effects of hypnotherapy on hay fever symptoms. The study of 66 volunteers with hay fever took place over two years and encompassed two hay fever seasons, and the subjects continued to take their normal allergy medications throughout.[8] After a year, during which one section of the volunteers were taught to practise self-hypnosis, it was found that they had fewer symptoms than the volunteers who had not practised self-hypnosis. The 'untrained' volunteers were then taught how to self-hypnotize during the second year, and they also reported an improvement in their symptoms. Most of the volunteers were also able to reduce their hay fever medication. Scientific checks were made of the volunteers' air-flow, and it was found that they could exhale more forcefully through their nose, even when exposed to substances that triggered their symptoms.

Professor Langewitz, who conducted the study, says that hypnosis could work by altering the speed of blood flow through the tissues in the nose, helping to alleviate stuffiness and congestion.

There are many anecdotal reports of improvements from using hypnotherapy, but experts generally state that there is not enough scientific evidence for this type of treatment to be promoted. It is definitely an area worthy of further research, and it is to be hoped this takes place in years to come.

Homeopathy

The homeopathic approach to medicine is holistic: the overall health of a person – physical, emotional and psychological – is assessed before treatment commences. The homeopathic belief is that the whole make-up of a person determines the disorders to which he or she is prone, and the symptoms that are likely to occur. Indeed, homeopaths profess that their remedies assist the body in its natural tendency to heal itself. A homeopath will ask you about your medical history and personality traits, then offer a remedy compatible with your symptoms as well as with your temperament and characteristics. Consequently, two individuals with the same disorder may be offered entirely different remedies.

Homeopathic remedies are derived from plant, mineral and animal substances, which are soaked in alcohol to extract the 'live' ingredients. This initial solution is then diluted many times, being vigorously shaken each time to add energy. Impurities are removed and the remaining solution made up into tablets, ointments, powders or suppositories. Low dilution remedies are used for severe symptoms while high dilution remedies are used for milder symptoms.

The homeopathic concept has, since antiquity, been that 'like cures like'. It is said that the full healing abilities of this type of remedy were first recognized in the early nineteenth century when the German doctor Samuel Hahnemann noticed that the herbal cure for malaria – which was based on an extract of cinchona bark (quinine) – actually produced symptoms of malaria. Further tests convinced him that the production of mild symptoms caused the body to fight the disease. He went on to successfully treat malaria patients with dilute doses of cinchona bark.

Each homeopathic remedy is first 'proved' by being taken by a healthy person – usually a volunteer homeopath – and the symptoms noted. This remedy is said to be capable of curing the same symptoms in an ill person. The whole idea of 'proving' and using homeopathic remedies can be difficult to comprehend, as it is exactly the opposite of how conventional medicines operate. For example, a hay fever patient with a very runny nose and watery eyes would be given a remedy that would produce these same symptoms in a non-hay fever sufferer. Conventional medicine, on the other hand, would provide something that stops the nose running and dries up the tear ducts.

Homeopaths claim that nowadays a remedy can be formulated to aid virtually every condition, including allergy disorders. Indeed, thousands of hay fever sufferers – plus the parents of young children with hay fever who would rather treat their offspring with a non-chemical therapy – are turning to homeopathy for symptom control and the chance of a reduced sensitivity to allergens. Homeopaths even state that their remedies can cure the condition.

Although such remedies are safe and non-addictive, occasionally the patient's symptoms may worsen briefly. This is known as a 'healing crisis' and is usually short-lived. It is actually a good indication that the remedy is working well.

A range of homeopathic remedies can be found in most high street chemists, while more specific ones are available from online homeopathic chemists (see Useful addresses at the back of this book for details of one such pharmacy). When self-prescribing, it is advisable to use the 30c potency. Below are some common remedies for particular hay fever symptoms:

- *Allium cepa* – For frequent and violent sneezing, a streaming nose with watery discharge, watery eyes, raw-feeling throat and nose and soreness beneath the nose and around the lips. Symptoms are worse in the morning and indoors.

- *Sabadilla* – For excessive nasal discharge, constant sneezing, stuffiness and the sensation of burning or severe itching in the nose, raw throat and palate. Cold sweats may be evident during the worst of the attack, and the person may obsessively think about his or her health situation. Just thinking about grasses and flowers can exacerbate symptoms.
- *Arsenicum iodatum* – For frequent sneezing and nasal discharge that may be either clear or thick and green. The discharge may be so continuous that it may seem hot and irritating, reddening the nose and nasal passages. There may also be shortness of breath, a hacking cough, hoarseness and a burning throat.
- *Belladonna* – For a throbbing headache, severe bouts of sneezing, a red, dry and hot face and a burning throat which can be relieved by drinking cool lemonade.
- *Arsen alb* – For a streaming nose, severe and painful sneezing with a burning mucus discharge which makes the upper lip sore.
- *Gelsemium* – For a blocked nose, hot flushed face, dizziness and drowsiness.
- *Euphrasia* – For a runny nose with a lot of sneezing and burning eyes which constantly itch and water. Euphrasia is also available as a tincture – in liquid solution form – which can be used as a soothing eye bath.
- *Wyethia* – For severe itching of the throat, nose and roof of the mouth (soft palate).
- *Pulsatilla* – For excessive thick white or yellow catarrh and frequent sneezing which eases in the open air.

If you have struggled with hay fever symptoms for several years and/ or your symptoms are severe, it is recommended that you make an appointment with a homeopath rather than self-prescribe. Commencing treatment before the hay fever season begins is said to make a real difference.

9

Hay fever and lifestyle

Anyone with more than the mildest of hay fever symptoms will say that it affects everything they do during the hay fever season. This chapter, therefore, offers advice on getting the most from all areas of your life.

Hay fever and education

Hay fever might not be classed as a serious condition, but it does cause many youngsters a great deal of distress – after all, trying to concentrate on the events of the English Civil War or the difference between adjectives and adverbs when your eyes are sore and your nose is dripping like a tap is hardly easy. However, it's the cumulative effect of several seasons of hay fever – that is, the fatigue, irritability and feelings of general malaise as well as the symptoms related to the upper respiratory tract – that can really affect a child's education.

There is nothing worse for a parent than seeing your child suffer. Another very real concern is the long-term effects of giving medications to a child. The fact is, though, that hay fever medications, when taken prior to symptoms commencing, can work so well at reducing symptoms that allergy experts claim that their very minimal risks are worth their numerous benefits. (See Chapter 5 for information on the medications on offer for hay fever.)

Hay fever and exams

After perhaps several years of tiredness and poor concentration in the classroom during the hay fever season – missed days off school, too, from time to time – a child or adolescent is hardly likely to absorb information in a way that is conducive to a favourable outcome where exams are concerned. In the UK there are plenty of important exams: SATS must be tackled at 7, 11 and 14 years of age, followed by GCSEs and A levels.

Added to this, the main time of year for taking school exams coincides with the peak season for the release of grass pollen – that is, from mid-May to the end of June. As a result, in examination rooms throughout the country (and indeed throughout the Western world), youngsters can be seen looking miserable and unwell, with cold-like symptoms that detract attention from the exam questions they are attempting to answer. Clearly, the effect on their achievements can be significant. Indeed, according to some studies around one in five children and adolescents sitting exams at any one time achieve worse grades than anticipated – and all due to hay fever.

An approximate 40 per cent of youngsters drop a grade between their mock and final exams, when the same grade or a grade up is expected. Of those taking a sedating antihistamine treatment, this figure is believed to rise to a staggering 70 per cent. It is a great shame that children and adolescents are still taking the older, sedating hay fever treatments, when improved, non-sedating ones are available, especially when the older ones have such an obvious detrimental effect. It is not only the attention span that is affected, but also working memory, speed, observation and carefulness, as discussed in Chapter 5. The youngsters concerned must find it difficult to stay awake during exams, let alone answer taxing questions. Fatigue, listlessness and reduced motivation are also problems. Moreover, a bad night's sleep due to sneezing and a streaming nose is likely to affect adversely performance in exams the next day.

University exam times are similar to those in school, so students with hay fever are just as likely to be hampered by their symptoms. Consequently, exam results might also not be what they should have been.

Controlling symptoms

Because severe hay fever can impinge so greatly on a youngster's education and ultimately their exam results, it is important that their symptoms are kept under control – and that non-sedating medication is used. Visits to the doctor's surgery well in advance of the start of the hay fever season are advised, to talk about symptom control, to enable the most appropriate medication to be prescribed. As described earlier in this book, some people are able to get their symptoms under control only by using a combination of treatments, while others, more fortunate, find that only one type of medication is required, which is perhaps available over-the-counter (without prescription) from your chemist.

If you really want to avoid giving medications to a child, consider trying the anti-allergy diet discussed in Chapter 7, using herbal remedies (see Chapter 6) and/or complementary therapies (see Chapter

8). Following the self-help advice in this book can also be enormously helpful. Children and adolescents with less severe symptoms may be able to manage by using the self-help guidelines alone, and perhaps by making a few adjustments to their diet.

Once hay fever symptoms are under control, you (or your child) will automatically begin sleeping better at night. As a result, you will wake up refreshed and find it much easier to concentrate on revision as well as exams.

Hay fever and work

Hay fever impinges on every area of your life, and that includes your working day. Those who find it a particular hardship are often in the following groups:

- People in the public eye, whose constant sneezing, eye-watering and nose-blowing make it difficult for them to interact effectively with other people. This group includes receptionists, shop assistants, publicans, teachers, actors, managers, doctors and nurses.
- People in leadership roles such as company directors and chief executives, who could perhaps feel that their authority was being undermined by constant sneezing and nose-wiping.
- People who are required to make vital decisions. Feeling tired, irritable and having the constant distraction of nose, eye and throat-related symptoms can make it difficult to balance the pros and cons of a problem and ultimately come to the best conclusion, or even worse, can make a wrong decision appear right until circumstances prove the opposite.
- People who drive for a living, or who need to drive in the course of their work. As hay fever can cause tiredness, distraction and poor judgement, it may actually be dangerous for a person with hay fever to be in charge of a motor vehicle.
- People who need to use their hands for their work. This group includes individuals employed in the construction industry, machine operatives, craftspeople, hairdressers, keyboard operators, gardeners, tele-sales staff, physiotherapists and musicians.

In order to function safely and effectively, people in these types of occupations need to take steps to control their symptoms, in ways discussed in this book. If, realistically, this requires a visit to your doctor, don't hesitate to go.

Hay fever and leisure activities

People with hay fever deserve to have just as much fun and enjoyment in their leisure time as anyone else. If you prefer energetic activities such as tennis, badminton, five-a-side football, basketball, netball and volleyball, hay fever shouldn't cause you to have to give them up during the peak season for hay fever – although you may have to use indoor sports facilities as an alternative.

If you participate in a sport that is generally only played outdoors – rugby, cricket or soccer, for example – you may have no choice but to forgo it for a few weeks, although there is every chance that you will be able to control your symptoms by using the most appropriate hay fever medications and taking heed of the advice in this book. Some people will be able to control their symptoms effectively enough to indulge in that twice-weekly game of football, while others with more severe symptoms may not be so fortunate and have to abandon the activity until they are feeling better.

Changing your leisure-time activities

If you have to temporarily abandon a certain outdoor activity, it's always tempting to sit at home feeling thoroughly miserable. Remember that there may be other activities you will enjoy equally, and perhaps find as pleasing and rewarding as the one you have had to put aside. Of course, certain sports such as cricket are played only during the hay fever season, and those passionate about participating can easily become depressed when they have to give them up.

You may have been selected to play in a prestigious team and have had no choice but to refuse your place. Such an outcome may not only be a real loss to your teammates and supporters, but also soul-destroying for you yourself. In instances such as this, it's worth impressing on your doctor how very important to you the particular activity is. You may then be referred to an allergy specialist, which will make it more likely that a treatment that works for you is found.

If swapping one activity for another is no real hardship for you, take advantage of the many indoor sports centres and activities. Or go swimming at your local baths. Swimming in the sea is also an option, if that's possible, as there is unlikely to be pollen circulating in the air over the sea.

Indoor hobbies

Your ability to do indoor hobbies, such as tapestry, knitting, sketching, model-making and craftwork, where you need to use your hands, can be impeded by your hay fever. Frequently wiping your nose and eyes can interfere dramatically with your concentration too, and you may find it impossible to make progress. Once again, seek your doctor's advice about the most appropriate treatments, and follow the advice in this book. If your hay fever is bad even when you are indoors, take particular heed of the self-help advice on pages 62–6.

Gardening

If you love gardening and your hay fever medications and/or self-help measures are at least partly controlling your symptoms, you may like to create a hay fever-friendly garden. You can do most of your work on the garden in March, which is before the start of the hay fever season for most people.

The following tips can make working in the garden more tolerable:

- Prior to going outdoors, check the daily pollen count for your area. If the signs are that it's going to be a high pollen count day, think of gardening another time.
- Spray a fine mist of water over the garden with the hose to dampen down pollen in the air.
- Use spectacles or wraparound sunglasses while gardening to keep pollen out of your eyes. Consider wearing a mask too, to protect your mouth.
- Keep your house doors and windows closed while you are outdoors.
- To keep pollen out of your hair, wear a hat when gardening. Whether or not you do so, brush your hair in your porch or other enclosed entrance area, if you have one, before coming indoors, otherwise put a comb in your pocket before going outside and pull it through your hair prior to coming back inside.
- Don't wear your gardening clothes around the house, as pollen sticks to fabrics.
- If your symptoms make it difficult to garden and there is no one else to do it, speak to your doctor about the possibility of temporarily increasing your medication while you prepare your 'anti-allergen' garden.
- Don't bring cut flowers indoors. If you are given some, shake them well outdoors before putting them in a vase (perhaps placing them in

an out-of-the-way area). It may be best, however, to ask people not to bring you flowers, explaining that they make your hay fever worse.

- There are two National Asthma Campaign low-allergen gardens. Try to visit at least one of them for lots of useful advice.

Plants

Steer clear of plants that release their pollen into the air; choose those that are pollinated by insects – this pollen is sticky and heavy, making it far less likely to become airborne. Most flowers with large petals are insect-pollinated, examples being clematis, iris and geranium. If you grow clematis and other climbing plants, keep them well away from your doors and windows. Pollen and dust can accumulate on the leaves and blow indoors.

Try to avoid growing flowering plants that are heavily scented, as this can temporarily worsen hay fever symptoms. These would include wisteria, jasmine, carnations, hyacinths and freesias. Among the best low-allergen annual plants are nigella, mimulus, antirrhinum, impatiens and eschscholzia.

Lawns

Lawns harbour numerous types of pollen, mould and dust, which all fly into the air when it is being mown. In place of a lawn you could use tiles, gravel mulch or one of the many types of attractive paving – or you could even use synthetic grass matting. These alternatives have the added advantage of being easier to maintain than grass. However, if you don't have a choice and must stick with a lawn, ask someone else to mow it, keeping the house doors and windows firmly closed beforehand and for several hours afterwards. Cylinder mowers cause less pollen and dust to fly into the air.

Shrubs

Shrubs are usually insect-pollinated and shouldn't cause a problem, and they are also quite easy to maintain. Think of using shrubs instead of traditional hedges to edge the boundaries of your land, but don't choose heavily scented ones – again, as with scented flowering plants, this can aggravate your symptoms.

If you want to try planting a herbaceous border, use low-allergy plants such as tiarella, viola, veronica, acanthus, aquilegia, pulmonaria, hosta, iris, campanula, delphinium, saxifrage, hemerocallis and geum perennial geranium.

Weeds

When you are weeding the garden your face is nearer the ground, and this allows airborne pollen to easily enter your nose and mouth. Low-allergen ground-cover plants can suppress weed growth, however – examples being ajuga, lamium, vinca and hostas. It's also a good idea to cover any patches of bare earth with gravel mulch as this can discourage weed growth.

Compost heap

The rotting vegetation in a compost heap is invariably full of mould, so it is best not to have one. Wrap up your waste vegetation in plastic bags and remove them from the garden. Avoid purchasing garden compost, too, as this can also harbour mould.

Water features and ponds

If you love the sound of running water and are considering a water feature, don't buy a fountain, as falling water generates air currents, which make pollen and dust rise into the air. Choose a smooth-running waterfall as this is less likely to create extra movement of air.

Most pond plants are not irritants, with the exception of the arum lily.

Pot plants

In a hay fever-friendly garden it is safe to have plants in pots. Don't bring them indoors in winter, though, as spores from moulds in the soil are released by the warmth of the house.

USA

American Academy of Allergy, Asthma and Immunology (Pollen and Mould Counts)
555 East Wells Street, Suite 1100
Milwaukee
Wisconsin 53202-3823
USA
Tel.: 414 272 6071
Website: www.aaaai.org
Email: info@aaaai.org

This is a membership-led organization giving information and advice about allergic disease, as well as the current pollen and mould counts for specific areas in the USA.

American College of Allergy, Asthma and Immunology
85 West Algonquin Road, Suite 550
Arlington Heights
Illinois 60005
Website: www.acaai.org
Email: mail@acaai.org

This is purely a web service giving information and advice about allergic disease. There is no facility for telephone contact.

National Institute of Allergy and Infectious Diseases
NIAID Office of Communications and Government Relations
6610 Rockledge Drive
MSC 6612
thesda
20892-6612

301 496 5717 (local number) or 866 284 4107 (toll free)
te: www3.niaid.nih.gov
via the website

nization provides the latest news and information about allergy
ious diseases.

Useful addresses

UK

Allergy UK
3 White Oak Square
London Road
Swanley
Kent BR8 7AG
Helpline: 01322 619868
Website: www.allergyuk.org
Email: info@allergyuk.org

This national charity aims to increase awareness of allergic disease, help people to manage their allergies, raise funds for allergy research and provide training for healthcare professionals including doctors, nurses, dietitians and pharmacists. Allergy UK is now the working title of the British Allergy Foundation.

Asthma UK
Summit House
70 Wilson Street
London EC2A 2DB
Tel.: 020 7786 4900 (switchboard)
Helpline: 08457 01 02 03 (Mondays to Fridays, 9 a.m. to 5 p.m.)
Website: www.asthma.org.uk
Email: info@asthma.org.uk

Asthma UK endeavours to increase public awareness of asthma and raise funds for research into the condition. It offers excellent information and advice for its members, together with a quarterly magazine which is full of the latest news and research from the world of asthma.

BBC Weather Centre
Website: bbc.co.uk/weather/pollen/index.shtml (for the daily pollen count)

This is a website giving details of local weather conditions, the daily pollen count, and information about climate change.

BioCare Ltd
Lakeside
180 Lifford Lane
Kings Norton
Birmingham B30 3NU
Tel.: 0121 433 3727
Website: www.biocare.co.uk
Email: sales@biocare.co.uk

This is a recommended supplier of healthcare products, including a nutritional supplement which helps to combat adrenal exhaustion.

Goodness Direct
South March
Daventry
Northants NN11 4PH
Tel.: 0871 871 6611
Website: www.goodnessdirect.co.uk
Email: info@goodnessdirect.co.uk

Many of the herbal supplements recommended for the treatment of hay fever are available from this company, including aloe vera juice, feverfew, echinacea, garlic, sage and goldenseal.

The Healthy House
The Old Co-op
Lower Street
Ruscombe
Stroud
Gloucestershire GL6 6BU
Tel.: 0845 450 5950
Website: www.healthy-house.co.uk
Email: info@healthy-house.co.uk

This mail-order business supplies products to people with allergies; they sell a wide range of allergy-related items such as pollen masks, air purifiers, ionizers and dust-mite-proof bedding.

Helios Homeopathic Pharmacy
97 Camden Road
Tunbridge Wells
Kent TN1 2QR
Tel.: 01892 536393
Website: www.helios.co.uk
Email: contact is via the website

Specific homeopathic remedies can be ordered through this website.

UK National Pollen and Aerobiology Research Unit (NPARU)
Website: www.pollenuk.co.uk

The NPARU is the main provider of pollen forecasts, fungal spore forecasts and pollen data for the UK.

Australia

The Asthma Foundation of Victoria
491–495 King Street
West Melbourne 3003
Victoria
Australia
Tel.: 03 9326 7088 or 1800 645 130 (toll free)
Website: www.asthma.org.au
Email: advice@asthma.org.au

This foundation gives information, advice and the latest resear

New Zealand

Allergy New Zealand
Website: www.allergy.org.nz
Email: via the website

The aim of this website is to provide sup'
ferers of allergic disease.

References

1 S. Gilardi et al., 'A prospective study in Locarno. (German) Schweizer-ische Medizinische Wochenschrift', *Journal Suisse de Medecine*, 1994, 124 (42): 1841–7.
2 P.J. Lachmann et al., *Clinical Aspects of Immunology*, Oxford: Blackwell Scientific, 5th edn, 1993.
3 N. E. Eriksson et al., 'Food sensitivity reported by patients with asthma and hay fever: a relationship between food sensitivity and birch pollen-allergy and between food sensitivity and acetylsalicylic acid intolerance', *Allergy*, 1978, 33 (4): 189–96.
4 J. F. Florido-Lopez et al., 'Allergy to natural honeys and chamomile tea', *International Archives of Allergy and Immunology*, 1994, 108 (2): 170–4.
5 P. Cullinan et al., 'Early prescription of antibiotics and the risk of allergic disease in adults: a cohort study', *Thorax*, 2004, 59(1): 11–15.
6 I. S. Farooqui et al., 'Early childhood infection and atopic disorder', *Thorax*, 1998, 53: 927–32.
7 M. Thomas et al., 'Early life antibiotic exposure and subsequent risk of asthma: a case control study', *Thorax*, 2003, 58: iii67.
8 W. Langewitz et al., 'The effect of self-hypnosis on hay fever symptoms: a randomized controlled intervention study', *Psychotherapy Psychosomatics*, 2005, 74: 165–72.

Index